FRESHWATER HERITAGE

A History of Sail on the Great Lakes, 1670-1918

DON BAMFORD

Foreword by Maurice Smith

NATURAL HERITAGE BOOKS
A MEMBER OF THE DUNDURN GROUP
TORONTO

Published by Natural Heritage Books
A Member of The Dundurn Group
3 Church Street, Suite 500
Toronto, Ontario, M5E 1M2, Canada
www.dundurn.com

Library and Archives Canada Cataloguing in Publication

Bamford, Don
Freshwater heritage : a history of sail on the Great Lakes, 1670-1918 / Don Bamford ; foreword by Maurice Smith.

Includes bibliographical references and index.
ISBN 978-1-897045-20-6

1. Great Lakes (North America)— Navigation — History. 2. Sailing ships — Great Lakes (North America)— History. 3. Shipbuilding — Great Lakes Region (North America)— History. 4. Shipbuilding — Ontario — History. 5. Shipping — Great Lakes (North America)— History. 6. Canada — History — War of 1812 — Naval operations. I. Title.

HE635.Z7G74 2007   386'.509713   C2007-900194-7

1   2   3   4   5   11   10   09   08   07

Front Cover: *The St. Lawrence*, O.K. Schenk, artist; back cover: *The Alvin M. Clark*, Charles L. Peterson, artist. All original paintings and all sketches, maps and photographs are courtesy of the author unless otherwise indicated.

Cover and text design by Sari Naworynski
Edited by Paul Carroll and Jane Gibson
Printed and bound in Canada by Hignell Book Printing of Winnipeg

Care has been taken to trace the ownership of copyright material used in this book. The author and the publisher welcome any information enabling them to rectify any references or credits in subsequent editions.

J. Kirk Howard, President

We acknowledge the support of the Canada Council for the Arts and the Ontario Arts Council for our publishing program. We also acknowledge the financial support of the Government of Canada through the Book Publishing Industry Development Program and The Association for the Export of Canadian Books and the Government of Canada through the Ontario Book Publishers Tax Credit Program and the Ontario Media Development Corporation.

As long as I can remember, I have been addicted to books.
My life's partner, Jean, has been very patient but frequently promised
to put a book in my hands when I am "laid to rest."
Unfortunately she preceded me.

To Jean, my first mate, I offer this historical tribute to her memory.
And to the authors who have come before me,
I humbly dedicate this book.

TABLE OF CONTENTS

Acknowledgements

I ACKNOWLEDGE A GREAT DEBT to the earlier writers who not only whetted my appetite by their own works, but also made my own search much easier by providing extensive bibliographies for their works. Prominent among them were Father Louis Hennepin, George Cuthbertson, C.H.J. Snider, President Theodore Roosevelt, Captain H.C. Inches, Howard Chapelle and many, many more. The list goes on and on. A new surge of interest, at least on the Canadian side of the International Border, seems to be occurring. Works by authors, Barry Gough, Robert Malcomson and Thomas Malcomson, Arthur B. Smith and others have appeared. An excellent maritime artist, Peter Rindlisbacher has also added his splendid visual works. He will undoubtedly be known as one of the best marine artists in the field. They all have brought me great pleasure.

Further, to gather much additional information, I visited and corresponded with museums and historical societies all around the lakes and across the eastern seaboard of the United States. To these and similar societies in England, France, Holland and the Scandinavian countries, I owe much gratitude for their assistance.

To my long time friend, counsellor and fellow enthusiast of history and sailing, Paul Carroll, without whose influence and input this book would probably still be a "work in progress" I owe a great debt. His knowledge of writing proper English, word processing and publishing procedures is far superior to mine and he has corrected many of my errors and omissions. For any that remain, I take full responsibility.

I also thank those who assisted in locating visuals and additional background information: Paul Adanthwaite, Archives &

Collections Society, Picton, Ontario; Ian Bell, Port Dover Harbour Museum, Port Dover, Ontario; Ann-Marie Collins, Bruce County Archives, Bruce County Museum & Cultural Centre, Southampton, Ontario; Rob Cotton, Grey Bruce Image Archives, Owen Sound, Ontario; Pat Hamilton and Jeremy Allin, Huron County Museum, Goderich, Ontario, and Peter White of Toronto for sharing his memorabilia on the *Bruno*. I also thank Heidi Hoffman and James Sommerville for providing maps and sketches.

In my earlier texts, and for all of my published articles, I have held the sole responsibility for editing. The challenge to review the manuscript, to make it more readable and to correct the inimitable errors was mine and mine alone. In the case of this current work, however, I have been blessed to have the assistance of a stalwart editor, Jane Gibson, who has worked diligently to improve my manuscript. Albeit a subject quite foreign to her broad experience with Canadian heritage, she has persevered. Her suggestions, her questions and her offers to help make the text more presentable to the general readership for whom this work is intended, and her work has been of inestimable value. I am grateful for her tireless assistance.

Foreword

This book is written from the perspective of a author who has been to sea. He brings to the pages that follow an intimate understanding of the Lakes because he has sailed on all of them, anchored in their bays and like all experienced sailors, had close calls in the dark of night when fierce winds and tumbling waves are unforgiving.

With a few exceptions, Don's perspective is from the point of view of those sailors, scholars and authors who lived closer to the age of sail. Those sources have been well read and analyzed by Donald and the result is thoughtful good read. This book may not, as he says with great respect, "enamour the skilled and the knowledgeable writers of pure and scholarly Canadian history." Don's intent is to enlighten and entertain you in the spirit of his predecessor, G.A. Cuthbertson who wrote *Freshwater* in 1931.

This book may be the very catalyst you need to awaken a nascent interest in a subject that can easily become a passion.

MAURICE D. SMITH, KINGSTON, ONTARIO

Maurice D. Smith is the Curator Emeritus of the Marine Museum of the Great Lakes at Kingston. Prior to his museum career he sailed at sea and on the Great Lakes as captain of the sailing vessel *Pathfinder*, one of two Toronto Brigantine vessels. He is the author of *Steamboats on the Lakes*, published by James Lorimer & Company in 2005.

Prologue

Don Bamford is a talented and knowledgeable seaman. Largely self-educated in matters about ships and the sea, he has applied the expertise of his profession to a lifelong love of messing about with boats, with navigation and with the history of sail, sailors and their energizing adventures on the water. As a former builder of boats, he has applied the theories of engineering and construction, albeit with contemporary materials, to his pastime. He added a two-foot section to his last pleasure yacht, *Foudroyant*, and converted her from a ketch to a yawl.

"Better to ride the ocean waves, and to tend to herself," I am sure he would say.

My wife Mary and I first met Don as a dockside friend at the Maitland Valley Marina in Goderich many years ago, when we shared a two-boat well at the local yacht basin. We enjoyed his knowledge, garnered his advice and sought his expertise, as we, with a young family, learned our own ropes, so to speak in our then-recent and growing adventures with sailing. Some of our acquaintances found him to be a bit crusty. A real old salt in the classic tradition, one might say. He looked the part, too, with a bushy white beard, a tousled mop of wiry white on top, which his loving wife Jean tended, from time-to-time, as Don might permit.

Don and Jean would invite us over for the five o'clock cocktail hour, and we would gam together, for longer it seemed than we should. We soon learned that Don had been writing in Canadian and American yachting journals and the popular boating magazines for several years. We were introduced to his first book, *Enjoying Cruising*

Under Sail, first published in 1978, and endorsed by the Canadian Yachting Association as recommended reading for any "sailor who wishes to cruise safely and competently and achieve the maximum return of pleasure for all."

We were soon to become the subjects, incognito, for photographs in an article about rescuing and recovering a comatose crew member at sea when Don invited us over to assist with a regimen, using a sail, a block and tackle, along with a halyard to haul an unconscious body from the water on to the deck of his boat. I was the unconscious body. Fortunately, I did not have to be knocked over the side. The only imperative was that I jump willingly, clad in full dress and life jacket, into the frigid waters.

The photos were really quite remarkable. You would swear we were at open sea. Don was a remarkable photographer as well, you see. He was very skilled in this additional pastime, and was in great demand for many years for his illustrated talks about his many sailing adventures. Mary and I were pleased to become active, yet unnamed, participants in one more of the literally hundreds of magazine articles that Don was to see published before the end of his ambitious sailing pursuits. Imagine my pride as the poor drowned sailor in the photos for a yachting safety feature in magazines published across Canada, the USA, and the UK!

Don was also an historian. On the Great Lakes, after he studied about the life and times of a particular maritime adventurer, or had his interest pricked about some vessel's misadventure on one of the lakes, you would find him setting off with his devoted partner and first mate, Jean, to seek out those same passages and the shorelines to understand even further the course of events of a given misfortune. He would sail the equivalent routes, as much as they were known. He would study options and alternatives to answer questions about mysterious disappearances. He would attempt to discover first-hand, the not-so-apparent clues to resolve the many unknowns.

Don was a religious man. He has been derived of a strong Methodist parentage, his father a member of that clergy. He has studied the Bible in considerable depth. Although he does not say so, I know that he has been fascinated with the sailing voyages of St. Paul at the time of Christ. And, it is clear to me that he has also followed those voyages during his retirement year of winter-sailing excursions on his beloved *Foudroyant*. Jean confided those same sentiments as we joined her and Don on a sailing junket in the northern Aegean, to visit Kavala, in northern Greece, and to climb through the ruins of Philippi, the site of the first Christian church in Europe.

He cast free his lines from the docks at the Goderich marina shortly after his retirement, and sailed away for the next fifteen years, and logged some fifteen thousand nautical miles. To get himself ready for ocean crossing while at Goderich, he would set out around dusk to single-hand across to Michigan on a Friday evening, and then sail back to Goderich on Saturday night.

"Sailing alone at night was no different than sailing in daylight," he declared, "except that it was dark."

He travelled south first, into the Caribbean, then across the Atlantic Ocean, circumnavigating the British Isles, crossing the rivers and canals of Europe on two occasions, touring much of the Mediterranean, and sought out shores within the forbidden territories of the Black Sea. He was uninvited by some not-so-friendly Russian officers at Odessa and required to leave the shores forthwith without landing.

In the Aegean Sea, he followed the theoretical routes of St. Paul, toured the sea-battle routes of Alexander the Great, thence returning north to inspect the Scandinavian shores, make a further incursion to Russia, this time to St. Petersburg. Finally, he returned to Cornwall and Falmouth Harbour as ill health and failing vision dictated that his sailing times had reached an end.

Now, at age 87, he is completing the final editing of his major manuscript to tie his learnings together. It is the third full book on some aspect of sailing. (The second was a comprehensive treatise entitled *Anchoring*, a text that continues to serve as a valuable resource for serious cruisers.)

Freshwater Heritage has been a passionate labour of love. It has taken a full generation of time to complete, time that could not be interrupted by sailing. In the course of its completion, Don has for-gotten more than most of us will ever remember on the subject. Perhaps he can be forgiven if he has not fully complied with the tech-nical aspects of completely documenting his notes, or verifying each and every one of his references. He is a noble man who is worthy of our honour and respect. His integrity speaks volumes for his subject.

The History of Sail on the Great Lakes is a necessary work "for the ordinary man." Its manner of presentation is in the informal style of C.H. Jeremiah Snider, one of Canada's most prolific writers of mar-itime history, who became the respected managing editor of the *Toronto Evening Telegram*. Don's commitment to tell this important story, in a readable and popular format, is needed. It should never be taken to deride the more formal and scholarly works of pure history. Don could never undertake such disrespect.

We credit Don Bamford with the inspiration to extend our own sailing quests, well beyond the Great Lakes at this time. We presently winter in the waters of the Bahamas on our sailing sloop, the *SolSean*. Even now as he counsels us to acquire our own levels of comfort before continuing this adventure, we look eagerly to farther shores, perhaps to Cuba and the nether islands beyond.

Some Notes about the Manner of Presentation

Some readers may be confused by apparent discrepancies in spelling throughout the manuscript. Don has used our familiar Canadian forms of spelling as might be found in the Canadian Oxford Dictionary for most of the language. However, he has retained the American spelling for place names found within the USA and for vessels and harbours flying the American flag. He has also honoured the spelling conventions found within quotations by individuals and phraseology taken from the various historical sources he has used throughout his manuscript.

Imperial measure has been retained, as it was the convention of the period for which this document was written. Gender specific lan-guage, as required for the conveyance of the male-prevalent callings, careers and military related activities, has also been retained. Where appropriate, efforts have been made, outside of direct quotations, to use contemporary language conventions that might be described as more politically correct for these times in the 21st century.

The reader will see Chippewa and Chippawa, both used correctly, as they were in the historical settings cited. And yes, there was a Presque Isle and there was also a Presqu'île.

For ease of identification, the names of all sailing vessels have been *italicized*.

PAUL CARROLL
Goderich, Ontario

Introduction

I DO NOT KNOW WHAT STARTED MY INTEREST in the history of sail on the Great Lakes. I had little interest in history during my early education. My teachers, should any survive, would corroborate this fact. Even though I do not know how the interest started, I do know how fascinating the subject became to me. The actors in these various maritime historic events awakened in a way my history teachers never imagined they could. What my instructors required me to learn by rote — dates, places, names, losers and winners — I now learned through close and vivid intellectual acquaintance with the participants. Further, some of the early adventurers I came to know would have been total strangers to those who tried to drive history into me, and into the thick skulls of other youngsters in their classes.

I also learned that perspectives about our history depend upon who is writing it. Two writers covering the same war or battle wrote in such a way that one might believe they were describing entirely different events. As my research proceeded, mainly in Chicago, where I lived for several years, in Toronto, Ottawa, and England and, as I dug deeper and deeper, I felt a need to bring the stories to public attention as best I could, albeit with my limited ability.

I have been blessed with opportunities to sail extensively on the Great Lakes in my own boat. All the lakes were my playground and it was not hard to imagine these past explorers, be they now described as heroes or villains. In some cases, I followed the routes of these early adventurers for parts of their journeys. How intriguing it was to explore the routes, the passageways and the harbours used by some of these brave and daring sailors.

My profession, once my formal education was complete, included engineering and construction, theory, practice and technology. I have been fascinated by the methods of manufacture, the techniques, the tools, the materials, and most of all, the accomplishments of marine artisans. The work of the artificers of the 17th, 18th and 19th centuries was remarkable. Their achievements were astonishing. Their work was undertaken in an environment difficult to imagine today. By and large, the skills and expertise of that period have been lost, but it has been important to me to try to bring them back to life, at least in the written word.

Over the years, and continuing today, there have been many books published on early sailing craft. They include scholarly works for the specialist, coffee-table books and books for the general reader. However, the broad topic of "sail" on the Great Lakes has been neglected for over seventy years. The last good book on my subject was by George A. Cuthbertson in 1931. It has long since become a collector's item.

There is a need to remember the early exploits and accomplishments related to the evolution of sail on the Great Lakes. The ways of life, the arts and skills of those who laid the foundations for our history must be committed to paper for the benefit of those who have already forgotten, if indeed they ever knew of these times. Perhaps I will inspire a few others to delve more deeply and to learn even more.

I commissioned the paintings by C.L. Peterson and by O.Z. Schenk. Both these men are recognized artists of the highest order, but, equally important, both have a love for sailing, for the sea, and for accuracy in the rendition of a ship's features, hull and rigging, keel to masthead. Further, both have first-hand knowledge of how a vessel rides the waves, throws spray and, in all respects, how she behaves and how she appears in her natural element. Both artists, as personal friends, encouraged me in this endeavour.

The painting of a timber drogher was given to me by my wife, Jean, in 1972 and was my first introduction to Charles (Chick) Peterson. If this gift was not the actual spark, at least it provided the fuel for my interest in the topic. The others he painted for me were based on my research in old texts and articles on the architecture and construction of early vessels.

The rendition of the *St. Lawrence* by Ozzie Schenk was based on similar research, plus visits to museums, in particular the National Maritime Museum in Greenwich, England. They kindly supplied me with a copy of the original "as built draught," or drawing, of the ship. Ozzie Schenk also did his own research and both of us were assisted by members of "The Provincial Marine of 1812," who were a great help. Of course, the artists themselves contributed much from their personal knowledge of the subjects.

I sent a copy of the painting to the National Maritime Museum in Greenwich and they concurred that the rendition was reasonably anatomically accurate, except that "Perhaps the bowsprit should be steeved a bit more steeply."

I believe that all these pictures represent very accurately what these ships might have looked like, which is all I wanted to do. Their exact appearance will never be known and I do not claim the paintings to be absolutely authentic. The paintings by Chick Peterson and Ozzie Schenk are part of the author's collection.

Churchill is credited with writing, "History is one damn thing after another." I did not set out to write a scholarly book for academics, but rather, one that would make a few of these "damn things" entertaining for the majority of peoples living in the Great Lakes basin. As a matter of fact, I hope that these words will motivate anyone anywhere who may have an interest in sail or sailing. May these words inspire them to read further. Hence, I have included an extensive bibliography.

My mandate is to write about the ships, their builders, their methods, their supply and personnel problems; and what life was like in the shipyards and on board. This theme does not include the politics, the military strategies, or the battles, except in so far as an explanation of these may help clarify my main subject, and, it is hoped, better inform the reader regarding the events.

As a matter of fact, in my efforts to interpret and to condense important historical events, there may have been some unintended latitude taken to convey an impression, which rightly, might have been further explored. This informal approach will surely not enamour the skilled and the knowledgeable writers of pure and scholarly Canadian history. It is not my intent to offend, nor is it my desire to misstate any events from our past. But I do wish to communicate a meaningful sense of the history of sail, as it may have been affected by historical events as they unfolded. There are many fine sources of such pure histories. To those outstanding pieces of work, I refer any reader for whom my words may have transgressed the acceptable. My intent is to provide a popular history for common use.

The subject of shipbuilding in established "old world" shipyards has been covered by European writers, but, to my knowledge, shipbuilding in a wilderness setting has never been described by writers in Europe, nor in any detail in North America by any author on this continent. Such is my task.

So much for our "freshwater heritage." It is important that its substance be passed on to our children.

DON BAMFORD
London, Ontario
February 2007

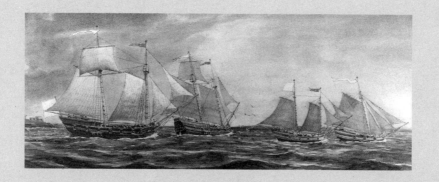

PART ONE

The Era of French Control on the Great Lakes, 1678–1760

"A people which take no pride in the noble achievements of remote ancestors will never achieve anything worthy to be remembered with pride by remote descendents." – Macaulay

"It is opportune to look back on old times and to contemplate our fathers." – Sir Thomas Browne

The French Fleet of 1757, Captain Pierre Bouchard de la Broquerie, artist.
He was stationed at Fort Frontenac and dated the drawing 1757.
Courtesy of the Toronto Reference Library (TRL) T15213.

CHAPTER 1

The Beginning of Sail on Lake Ontario, 1678

I HAVE FOUND NO RECORD OF the use of sail by the Aboriginals on the Great Lakes, nor of the use of sail on the Eastern Seaboard before the arrival of the Europeans. If there had been any, surely it would have been mentioned in the writings of early explorers, settlers and missionaries. It seems that the First Nations peoples were not acquainted with the art of sailing, though their bark canoes were the best of all forms of the canoe family to be found anywhere in the sixteenth and seventeenth centuries. It is quite probable that early explorers such as Champlain, Brûlé, Radisson, Des Grosseilliers and Rosenboom (an early Dutch explorer of that same era) and their followers used makeshift sails of skins or blankets. The Native North Americans seem to have picked up the idea, though only in rudimentary fashion and for downwind sailing.

Father Louis Hennepin, (May 12, 1626–c.1705), baptized Antoine, was a Catholic priest and missionary of the Franciscan Récollet Order and an explorer of the interior of North America. Although Hennepin was born in Belgium, he became French in 1659, when Béthune, the town where he lived, was captured by the army of Louis XIV of France.

At the request of Louis XIV, the Récollets sent four missionaries to New France in May 1675, including Hennepin, accompanied by René Robert Cavalier, Sieur de la Salle. Three years later, Hennepin was ordered by his provincial superior to accompany La Salle on a voyage to explore the western part of New France.

Hennepin reported, "When the Wind is favourable they [the Indians] make use of little Sails made of birch bark, but thinner than that used to make the canoes, and they can expedite to a Miracle."¹ In the same paragraph he explains how the Europeans made use of linen cloth hoisted up a little mast. Pierre Pouchot, a French officer during the Seven Years War, wrote in his memoirs, "They add a mast, made of a piece of wood, and cross piece to serve as a yard, and their blankets serve them as sails."² This information, such as it is, is all I have found regarding the use of sail by the First Nations people.

The Aboriginals had developed their canoes to a high level of efficiency. They were well suited for their purpose. They were fast and very manoeuvrable and excellent for the rough waters of the countless streams and rivers that they had to navigate. The need to cross large bodies of water, such as coastal bays and the Great Lakes, was of much lesser importance. Sail would not have been practical in the waters they normally navigated. Not only would sails have been a nuisance, but they would also have created a serious impediment to fast portaging.

Moreover, the basic shape of the canoe was quite unsuitable for sailing in any direction other than downwind. These craft had no keel and were quite smooth on the bottom. Of course, some form of leeboards could have been added to act like a keel, which would have helped, but there is no record that this was ever tried. On top of that, as anyone knows who has tried canoeing, these craft are basically unstable and prone to capsize.

The first actual sailing craft were those to arrive at the coast from the mother countries, bringing explorers and settlers with them. Even the earliest settlements included shipwrights and others with knowledge of the arts and skills of shipbuilding as practised in the homeland. Such skills were commonplace in England, Holland,

France and Spain in the 16th and 17th centuries. The first recorded shipbuilding in America occurred when François du Pontgrave, an early French fur trader, launched two small sailing vessels, a barque and a shallop (an open rowing and sailing vessel built to carry cargo used for fishing, or just for travelling on the water) at Port Royal in 1606. Further south, shipbuilding started when the 32-ton *Virginia* was built at the mouth of the Kennebec River in New England (Maine) in 1607. She carried homesick and disillusioned immigrants back to England in 1608 and apparently made several voyages back and forth in subsequent years.

The Dutch in New Amsterdam[3] built a sailing vessel starting in 1615, the 45-foot *Onrust*. She explored the coastline of what is now Rhode Island, Connecticut and New Jersey, and journeyed up the Delaware Bay. Later, she carried a load of furs back to Holland. In 1631, the first "government ship," the *Blessings Of The Bay*, was built by English settlers of Massachusetts Bay. She was of 30 tons and used for fur trade along the coast and with the Dutch at New Amsterdam.

These vessels and others of the early settlers were built as occasion required, in clearings in the forest, near the coast. Proximity to timber was essential. Frequently the building site was some distance from the coast. Once ready, the vessels were then hauled across the snow (it was easier to pull the heavy weight in the winter snow or to haul them on rollers in summer months) by teams of oxen or horses and launched into some stream, ready for spring run off.

Shipbuilding was a casual affair at first. As an industry, it did not appear to start until around 1640. Prior to that time, shipwrights and carpenters were not brought out specifically for the purpose of shipyard work. The need for ships for the West Indian trade made the commercialization of the work necessary, and many small shipyards were established in New England and around Chesapeake Bay. By the turn of the century, there were thriving shipyards at the mouths of rivers in Maine, Connecticut, Massachusetts, New York and in Virginia, Pennsylvania and Maryland.

In French North America, in 1670, Jean Talon, Intendant of New France, established the first shipyard by the Charles River at

Quebec and built a 120-ton vessel. This was probably the largest ship to be constructed in America up to that time. Very little has been detailed about these early days of shipbuilding in North America, but it is safe to conclude that the ships were essentially similar to those built in the home countries in the same period. Furthermore, the tools and methods were close to identical to those of the homeland except in so far as was demanded by differences in species of wood and in supplies, in terrain and in weather. Undoubtedly, shortages of conventional materials, and especially of iron, required a great deal of innovation and ingenuity on the part of the builders.

Tools and methods did not change much in the several centuries preceding the application of mechanical power. Around 1796, steam saws were coming into use in England, preceded only slightly by saws driven from power derived from the waterwheel. Try, if you will, to visualize the problems faced in these early shipyards: no power, no buildings, green timber – still standing in the forest – uncooperative weather, unfriendly Natives, to name only a few.

Into this scene, in 1678, came La Salle to establish the first shipyard in the freshwater lakes, at Fort Frontenac, now Kingston, Ontario. The French had, in fact, been trading on the lakes for over 60 years, for there were fortunes being made in the fur trade. The Jesuits were busy in the area in their efforts to convert great numbers of the heathen Aboriginals to Christianity. There were a few scattered outposts, little more than shelter for the voyageur, and a few struggling missionary stations, but there had been very little effort at real settlement.

René-Robert Cavalier was born in Rouen in 1643, of wealthy and high-placed parents. He took the name Sieur de La Salle from the name of his parents' estate. La Salle was educated in a Jesuit College with the intent of giving his life to the work of the religious order. However, he proved too restless for this type of life and, after a brief career in the army of France, he took monies left to him on his father's death and sailed for Canada in 1666. As a result of his parting from the Order, he had a falling out with the Jesuits.

As a consequence of his high connections, he was given a tract of land in New France, a seigneury of which he became, in effect, a feudal owner. He in turn sublet the land to small farmers and settlers, erected a palisaded fort, trading house and dwelling. Dreaming of further explorations to the west, he named it "a la Chine," and eventually it developed into the present-day city of Lachine. At the time the prevailing idea was that a route existed through the Great Lakes, and possibly the Mississippi Valley, to the Eastern Sea and Cathay, a much coveted trading destination. From La Salle's perspective, a vessel built above the cataract at Niagara should be able to pursue this dream.

In 1669, La Salle obtained Letters Patent from the French King of France to proceed with his plans for exploration. However, no funds were forthcoming from the French government to support such an enterprise. Over the period from 1669 to 1671, he travelled by canoe through the Great Lakes and into Mississippi country, gaining first-hand knowledge of the waters his vessel would have to navigate.

At this time, all trading was officially controlled by the government of France, which licensed traders. All furs were required to be carried to Montreal or Quebec. Actually, however, there were many freebooters, financed by wealthy families in these towns or some even back in France, who traded with the Natives and sold their furs through the English traders and sometimes Dutch and German traders, in Albany or New Amsterdam.

La Salle, however, worked on the side of law and organized commerce according to the state requirements. He made many enemies among the financiers who backed these freebooters, and particularly among their wealthy patrons at home. It is believed that these men of popular repute and position in the colony of New France and in Paris were ultimately the cause of his downfall as he was interfering with the great financial benefits they were reaping from the illegal trade. Despite this opposition, La Salle was befriended by Count Frontenac,[4] the new governor general for New France (appointed in 1672). In 1674, La Salle went to France and was presented to court as Frontenac's protégé. As a result, he obtained from the Crown, the Seigneury of Fort Frontenac, then under construction at the site of present-day Kingston, Ontario. He was required to purchase the land for this seigneury as long as he agreed to improve it, to fortify it, to settle the land around it, to provide a church and to undertake other considerable expenses.

Further, he was elevated to the rank of the untitled nobles and therefore became governor of the adjacent lands and islands, subject to the orders of the governor general. His family and friends were overjoyed at this success. Among them was the Prince of Conti, a nobleman, financier, and friend of La Salle, who loaned him large sums of money for the purpose. However, La Salle's successes only served to further aggravate the merchants and others who were prospering from the illicit fur trade and did not sit well with the Jesuits with whom La Salle had long been at odds, but issues now included Frontenac's position of state superiority over religious authority.

La Salle prospered at his new base of operations, Fort Frontenac. In 1677, he made another visit to France, armed with recommendations from Governor General Frontenac. He won over the French Minister of Finance who agreed to endorse his plans and to acquire the royal charter and assent La Salle needed to carry out his great undertaking.[5] His goal was to open up the west for trade, to establish forts and trading posts, to apprehend illegal traders, to negotiate and trade with the Natives, and to develop navigation and shipping in the waters of the Great Lakes and the Mississippi River.

All this La Salle was to do at his own expense. He raised what capital he could from friends and relatives, but fell into the financial clutches of others less scrupulous, who caused him no end of trouble and eventually brought about his ruin. (It is reported that one man loaned him money at an interest rate of 40%.) La Salle immediately set about engaging shipwrights, including Moisé Hillaret, the man credited with the actual construction of the first sailing vessels on the lakes. He hired sawyers, carpenters, blacksmiths and labourers. He purchased all manner of supplies in France, which were dispatched to Canada in 1678. Plans were also drawn up for a vessel to be built on Lake Erie and another to be built on the Mississippi. Thus, it can be seen that the vessels were definitely continental in design and typical of the era.

On this visit to France, La Salle met and became close friends with Henry de Tonty, an Italian officer living in France because of political troubles in Italy. Tonty had lost a hand in the Sicilian Wars and wore an artificial appendage. This prosthesis he would use most effectually in encounters with the Natives, who treated him as "powerful medicine," and gave him the name of "Iron Hand." He became La Salle's lieutenant and proved ever reliable and loyal to him. To Tonty must go a very large part of the credit for La Salle's explorations and accomplishments.

Another character he met at this time was Luke the Dane, also known as Luc or Lucas. La Salle hired him to be his pilot for the expedition. Although Hennepin gives us little detail, La Salle hoped that Luc would become his right-hand man. He wanted him to assume major decision-making responsibilities and to be a competent leader with La Salle's advance parties and his sailing crews. Unfortunately, Luc showed incompetence as a pilot and an unfortunate degree of unreliability, and La Salle soon lost faith in Luc's ability to follow commands. Some writers put much of the blame on Luc, for example, for the loss of the *Griffon*. Perhaps this charge is not fair. As you encounter these details, you will have to draw your own conclusions.

La Salle, Tonty and La Motte de Lussiere, one of La Salle's recruits in France,[6] set out from La Rochelle on July 14, 1678, and arrived at Quebec two months later. Here they met Father Louis Hennepin, the Récollet priest who was eager to join the expedition to the Upper Lakes and to the Mississippi. Hennepin proved to be energetic and hardy, if somewhat unscrupulous After La Salle's death, he tried to appropriate some of the honors of the expedition to himself. He published two works, the first in 1683 in French, and the second in 1698 in English. The first is less detailed than the second, but seems more reliable. Both accounts are largely a plagiarism of La Salle's official communications to the French Minister of Marine in 1682. La Salle called Hennepin a great exaggerator, who wrote more in conformity with his own wishes than his knowledge. However, taking this observation into account and verifying the documentation with other records, where important facts need to be established, the Hennepin journal makes an fascinating story and is essentially very useful.

By November 8, 1678, the entire group – including shipwrights and others who had gone ahead – had all reached Fort Frontenac. Once there arrangements had to be made to get the men and supplies on to Lake Erie, since the shipyard of the *Griffon* was just above the Falls, an obstacle for their vessels.

At the same time a party of fifteen men was sent westward by canoe to trade with the Natives, collect furs and establish supply depots on Lake Michigan (then known as Lac des Illinois) in readiness for the arrival of the *Griffon*, as the vessel was to be named, upon completion of her construction. La Motte was instructed to build a stockaded warehouse at the mouth of the Niagara River and to cut a portage trail to a point above the Falls where a ship could be built. He was instructed then to proceed to build the ship. La Salle was to follow later with further supplies. On November 18, 1678, the shipbuilders set sail, some eighteen men in all, and proceeded from Fort Frontenac to Niagara. This was the first recorded voyage under sail in any of the Great Lakes.

Let us backtrack for a moment to discuss the sailing vessel used on this trip, and to identify others that had been built by La Salle at Fort Frontenac. Very little is known about the first vessels to ply Lake Ontario, not even their dimensions, nor even the dates of their launching. The names of only two survive, through the writings of Father Hennepin. They were the *Frontenac*, built 1673, and the *Kataraquay* (also called the *Cataraqui*), built 1674.

It is believed that one was larger than the others for it was referred to as the "…great barque of M. de La Salle." Even the number of ships, whether

A rendition of the probable appearance of the first sailing boats on the Great Lakes, built at Cataraqui by La Salle. The two foreground sails are primitive square sails. Sketch by C.H.J. Snider. Taken from Snider, *Tarry Breeks and Velvet Garters*, Toronto: Ryerson Press, 1958.

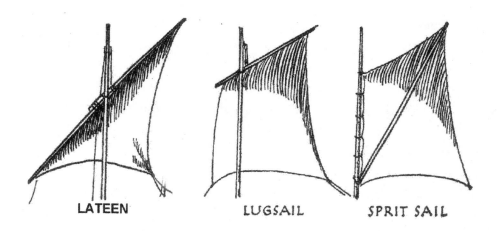

LATEEN   **LUGSAIL**   **SPRIT SAIL**

A sketch showing lateen, sprit and lug-sails. Snider's sketch of an early sailing vessel does not clarify this as the main sail is hidden.

three or four, is not definite. Hennepin writes that the one in which he, La Motte, and the sixteen labourers travelled, apparently the *Frontenac*, was small. According to Hennepin, it was some ten "tuns." They were all said to be brigantines.

"Tuns" were casks for wine or water, each carrying about 252 "wine gallons." The term has nothing to do with weight or displacement. Another word that is rarely heard today, "burthen" or "burden," means the number of "tuns" the vessel was designed to carry. If used today, the word "tons" refers to the weight of cargo or load capacity. As well, the word "brigantine," as used today, describes a specific sail and rigging plan for a vessel. But over the intervening three centuries, the term has described sail plans other than the modern brigantine as we know it. Even the earliest vessels, thus rigged, had too many sails to be practical for such a small craft.

Study of early treatises on naval architecture, particularly Frederik Henrik Chapman's *Architectura Navalis Mercatoria*, first published in 1775, would indicate that brigs were likely rigged with two masts on which were set sails, cut somewhat in the form of lugsails or spritsails, or even two lateen sails. These arrangements are simple to handle, permit quick furling in the event of a squall and perform reasonably well to windward. Certainly, these vessels were fitted out with oars as well as sail, for all sailors know better than to rely on the winds entirely.

Hennepin was not a sailor and may be forgiven if he used the wrong term. Many persons still have trouble properly identifying the sail plans seen today. However, it must be emphasized that all these conclusions are just conjecture, though it seems reasonable, as such rigs were in common usage for small coasting vessels of French, Flemish, Dutch and English construction. Typically, these would be about 45 feet in length with a 12 to 14-foot beam and have a depth of hold of some six feet from keel to deck. It is unlikely they were decorated with carvings as was customary for many of their European counterparts, nor painted except with locally-produced pine pitch.

A letter from Jean Baptiste Colbert, the great French Minister of Finance and the Colonies for Louis XIV, dated April 28, 1677, endorsing La Salle, said, "He has built four decked barques of which two are 25 tons, one of 30, and one of 40." Accommodation was very limited, probably restricted to a small, decked section in the bows and a tiny cabin under the quarterdeck at the stern, suited for perhaps four or five persons when sleeping. Possibly the largest boat was completely decked. The passengers would make shift in the hold or on deck as best they could. Cooking was probably accomplished on an open fire built upon the stone ballast in the hold.

Since such vessels were common in the mother countries, it is safe to guess that La Salle's men at Fort Frontenac would copy that with which they were familiar. The illustration here depicts a European vessel of the period. C.H.J. Snider illustrated his story of these vessels in *Tarry Breeks and Velvet Garters*[7] with a sketch that is a fair representation of how they may have appeared. Little more is known about this first shipbuilding enterprise or about the vessels built there.

We leave Lake Ontario now to pursue La Salle's adventures in shipbuilding above the Falls but will return later to see what happens on the lake. Thus, the scene is set and the purpose identified for the opening of navigation on the Upper Lakes with the building of and the maiden voyage of the *Griffon*. The facts and figures, as they apply to the people and their actions as outlined above, may be verified from historic documents. However, the details and specifications for La Salle's vessels are not documented.

CHAPTER 2

The Building of the *Griffon*, 1679

The bulk of the information on the building of the *Griffon*, and on its one and only voyage, comes from Father Hennepin's pen. It is unfortunate that he was not entirely reliable – bending the facts, as previously noted, to suit his own purposes, not an uncommon trait with some historians, however, one would expect better from a man of the cloth. Furthermore, his chronology of events leave much to be desired. Perhaps he can be forgiven for getting dates mixed up. His document, *A New Discovery of a Vast Country in America*, was published in England in 1698, some twelve years after the events. However, as it is the only narrative available, things will be put in proper order as best as possible. He left us very little in the way of specifications or details of the *Griffon*, and there has been much speculation by later writers. The material that I found most useful is contained in work by George Quimby in his book, *Indian Culture and European Trade Goods*.[1]

As noted earlier, La Motte and Hennepin, with 16 others in their party, set out from Fort Frontenac for Niagara on November 18, 1678, and attempted to proceed up Lake Ontario in boisterous Autumn weather. Hennepin wrote about this voyage and thus became the first of many hundreds to narrate sailing adventures there.

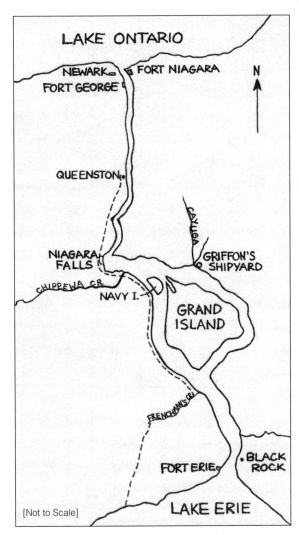

Sketch map of the Niagara River showing the site of the shipyard for building the Griffon *and the path followed when the gig of the* Charwell *was carried to Lake Erie. Map by Heidi Hoffman.*

It was a slow, uncomfortable passage and on the 26th of the month, most likely in cold and blustery weather, they put into the mouth of a river near the Indian town of Taiagon, considered to be at the Humber River, just west of present-day downtown Toronto. Here they traded with the Natives for corn, and, on December 5, had to chop away the ice to move out into the lake. Finally, after an arduous trip, they reached the Niagara River on the sixth of December, noted as a stormy night. It had been an extremely slow and uncomfortable voyage in an open boat in the late fall and winter weather. But they did score another first, for they had traded for corn at Taiagon and became the first of many grain carriers to ply the lake.

In the first two weeks of January, La Motte, Hennepin and five others made a diplomatic visit to the Seneca (Hennepin calls them "Iroquese") near present-day Rochester. On January 1, 1679, he preached to the Aboriginals in a small bark chapel. They negotiated for supplies and the blessing of their project, so that they might build their vessel above the Falls at the mouth of the Cayuga Creek (a small river in those days that empties into the Niagara just above the Falls on the American side) without harassment. While at the encampment, according to Hennepin, they witnessed the gruesome torture of a hapless Shawnee captive and observed subsequent grisly acts, which distressed the Europeans. Their "Embassie," as he referred to the visit, was generally unsuccessful, for they continued to have problems with the Natives and suffered considerable torment.

While this visit was progressing, their small vessel had already returned to Fort Frontenac for the others. La Motte began erecting his walled storehouse on the east bank of the Niagara River, a short distance upstream, near what is now Lewiston. He then commenced cutting a trail towards Lake Erie. The next voyage from Fort Frontenac to the Niagara River included La Salle and Tonty along with more workers and supplies. Luc the Dane acted as pilot. It is not clear whether the same boat was used or whether it was the "great barque of M. de La Salle."

In any event, December sailing was no more pleasant in 1679 than it is right now. In eight or nine days, they had gained only some 40 miles and were still on the Prince Edward shore, today's Prince Edward County by the Bay of Quinte. After grounding their vessel, yet getting off undamaged, they set course southwest for the mouth of the Genesee River on the south shore of Lake Ontario, today the location of Rochester, New York. La Salle wanted to negotiate with the Seneca for their support of his enterprise. They may have reached that destination and spent a week or so trading with the Natives, for on January 7 they were still held up on the south shore, not yet able to find their way to Niagara. They sat becalmed, and were unable to row through the crystallizing ice. La Salle and Tonty went ashore to hike, overland, to the shipyard above the Niagara cataract. La Salle appears to be unduly impatient, even irresponsible, in this act of leaving his valuable vessel and her cargo in the hands of Luc, whom he was now beginning to distrust even more than before.

As soon as La Salle and Tonty were out of sight, Luc and his companions anchored the vessel and clambered ashore to build a campfire and enjoy the relative comfort of sleeping in its warmth. They woke to a raging northerly gale. The boat was cast ashore and broke up, a total loss, though the crew managed to salvage part of her cargo. The site was named Cape Enragé or Mad Cape, its exact location unidentified. It must have been quite near the mouth of the Niagara River, for anchors and cables salvaged from the wreck were carried overland on the men's backs to the shipyard of the *Griffon*.

La Salle reached the construction site on January 20 and found the keel timbers roughed out from native white oak. The locale has been identified as being on the Cayuga Creek where it empties into the Niagara, an area now known as La Salle in present-day Niagara Falls, New York. Although La Salle also had grave doubts about the sincerity of La Motte as well as the loyalty of Luc, and in spite of considerable disaffection among the men, topped by unfriendliness from the local Natives, the work progressed. There is a letter in the Archives Judiciaires de Montréal, dated January 23, 1679, from La Salle at the shipyard to La Motte at Niagara, at the warehouse upstream from the mouth of the river. This letter is most enlightening, and throws some light on the sail plan of the *Griffon*:

> Also send along to the barque the sail canvas which is in the shack and please tell Lucas that the mainsail will have a spread of twenty-one feet and the mizaine sixteen feet. All he has to do is to give it to the men who are coming here. We can increase the sail area by using the two bonnets which always work very well.

Thus, it is known the *Griffon* was to have two masts.

La Motte seemed to lack physical endurance. He also suffered from some form of snowblindness or other eye affliction. He moved to Montreal about this time for treatment and drops out of the story. Fortunately, Master Shipwright Moisé Hillaret proved to be a most dependable leader for the construction project. Under his supervision, and with Tonty to maintain discipline, the work progressed well. La Salle, with several men, returned to the mouth of the Niagara and started the erection of blockhouses on the site of what became Fort Niagara. La Salle named the place Fort Conti in honour of his longtime friend and patron, but unfortunately most of it was burned later that winter and La Salle did not rebuild it.

La Salle was back at the shipyard on the 26th and, as Hennepin narrates, "The keel of the Ship and some of the Pieces being ready, M. La Salle sent the master Carpenter to desire me to drive in the first pin; but my Profession obliging me to decline that honour he did it himself." La Salle then:

> ...undertook his Journey afoot [to Fort Frontenac] over the snow, having no other Provisions but a little Sack of Indian corn, roasted, which fail'd him about two Days before he came to the Fort, which is above fourscore leagues distant from the place where he left us. However he got home safely with two Men and a Dog, who dragg'd his Baggage over the Ice or frozen Snow.

He spent most of the winter and early summer of 1679 travelling the 250 miles between Niagara, Fort Frontenac and Montreal, replenishing his lost supplies, placating his creditors and investors, and trading with the Natives. He does not appear to have returned to the shipyard until early August. To have travelled such distances, many of them by foot, is a most remarkable accomplishment.

On site at the shipyard, the problems faced by Moisé Hillaret, La Salle's appointed shipbuilder, and his thirty-four men were challenging. Only recently arrived from Europe, they were beset on all sides by Natives of very questionable friendship. For food, they had Indian corn, what whitefish they could catch, plus the ample culinary delights of locally hunted game. In this environment, they had to face the formidable task of building a great ship to sail the unknown seas.

There were neither horses nor oxen, so all the timbers had to be hewn within easy reach of the ship. The huge logs were dragged across the frozen, snow-covered earth to the sawpit where they were cut into timber and further shaped by the adze. The blacksmith shaped his bolts, spikes and other fittings at the forge. At this stage in history, various forms of saws, adzes, clamps, drills, chisels, mallets

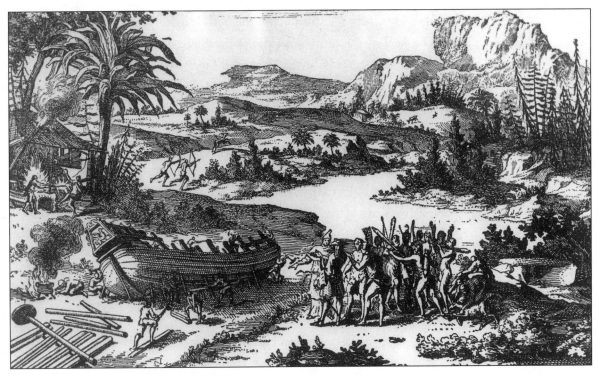

The Building of the Griffon, *1679*. Taken from the book A New Discovery of Vast Country in America *by Father Hennepin.*

and caulking tools, planes and moots (a tool of the plane family for making treenails or trunnels, a type of dowel fastener) plus the forge and anvil were in common usage in Europe. It can only be speculated that these many items had been conveyed to the site from the home-land. The difficulties appear almost insurmountable in today's envi-ronment. Without these very basic tools, the construction of such a ship would have been well nigh impossible in 1679.

The drawing by a Belgian artist (it appeared in Hennepin's book of 1698) does show a smithy at his forge, a worker using an adze, another using a mallet on deck and others using caulking tools.

Drills must have been available, for there was no other method of fastening together a vessel other than by wooden treenails. The "pins" used to hold keel and deadwood almost certainly would be iron drift-pins, undoubtedly brought from France, possibly partially forged on site. The great majority of fastenings would have been cut and shaped from local wood.

The planks were bent to proper shape through the use of steam-sweating boxes if they were available, or by soaking them for hours, then placing them over a fire. Screw clamps held them in place to the ribs and framework until they were secured by treenails, bolts or spikes. A study of the equipment in a shipwright's tool chest of the time discloses the fact that these old-time builders were equipped with most of the tools that are still in use today. All the modern carpenter can boast of today, in the nature of improved appliances, are the mechanical tools operated by electricity or by other power. The blacksmiths too, were well enough equipped in 1679, except that air for the forge had to be created by operating bellows instead of the electric-powered fan of the present day.

Undoubtedly, several kinds of wood were used in the construction of a typical vessel. White oak would have predominated as it was abundant in the vicinity. Rigging, anchors, sails, guns and other such supplies came from France, via Quebec, or Montreal and Fort Frontenac, as evidenced by Hennepin's chronicle and as documented in communications written by La Salle.

Some of the supplies were lost in the shipwreck at Mad Cape, but more than enough survived to complete the *Griffon* and to load it with iron for construction of a second vessel at Fort Crèvecoeur (heartbreak) near Peoria on the Illinois River. This vessel was never completed, but that is another story.

In spite of the many difficulties, our *Griffon* was launched early in May 1679. It was moored with two anchors out in the Niagara River near the building site, to await favourable winds, not being able to proceed any further against the current. In this location they were relatively safe from the Natives who had threatened to burn the ship. By July 4 she was completely rigged. Hennepin went back to Fort Frontenac to pick up two monks of his Order, and to advise La Salle that the *Griffon* was ready. The trip was made in one of the small barques that had sailed up that spring from Fort Frontenac to Niagara. Father Gabriel de la Ribourde and Father Zenobe Membre came back to the *Griffon* with Hennepin sometime around mid-July, and accompanied the expedition to Fort Crèvecoeur. La Salle rejoined his men in early August.

All the munitions of war, all the provisions and supplies were now transported over the portage from the lower Niagara to the *Griffon*, involving many a weary and painful journey. Even Father Gabriel, age 64, clambered up and scrambled down the escarpment several times, taking heavy loads to the shipyard. It required four persons to carry the heaviest anchor. The armament consisted of eight small cannon of iron and brass, three of which were described as "arquebuses-a-croc," that is to say, mounted on a swivel base. These small cannons could only be used to combat attacks from boarding parties of Natives, since they fired shot, perhaps the size of an orange, on a rather short range. In most cases, this weaponry fired a cloth or leather bag filled with grape shot.

Tonty and a party of five had gone ahead by canoe earlier, to trade for furs and to rendezvous at the mouth of the Detroit River. In the previous year, La Salle had sent fifteen men overland to the Green Bay area to trade with the Natives for furs. From Hennepin's narrative:

> Aug. 7 – A sharp breeze sprang up and the wind veering to the northeast and the Ship being well provided, we made all sail we could and with the help of twelve men who hauled from shore, overcame the rapidity of the current and contrary to the prediction of the pilot, got her up into Lake Erie.

And so the historic voyage begins!

CHAPTER 3

The Voyage of the *Griffon* and the Loss: Where is She Now?

ANYONE WHO HAS SAILED THE GREAT LAKES in a small boat, and is familiar with the excellent, modern charts, lighthouses, beacons and other aids to navigation (especially echo sounders to verify the depth, radio direction finders and the electronic wizard, the GPS or global positioning system) will consider the cruise relatively simple. Even so, it is not without some trepidation that the prudent sailor sets out, knowing that the weather can change quickly, and that the seas can suddenly become boisterous or worse. As one who has sailed from one end of the Great Lakes to the other, including passages made on both Lakes Michigan and Superior, known to be more treacherous, I can readily recognize the problems faced by the adventurers in the *Griffon* without so much as any navigation chart at all. That they ever made it from the Niagara River to Green Bay, Wisconsin, unaided, is a miracle in itself. But they accomplished this remarkable feat – and without mishap.

Hennepin's narrative is most intriguing. Those of you who are sailors will read between the lines. Just as might happen in our own experiences, there were breakdowns in crew relationships. Surviving a trip with 34 people together in a small boat for 26 days with no mutiny or outright fighting is another miracle.

Actually, La Salle felt it necessary to take over twice from Luc when he lost all confidence in his pilot, but it seems the two never came to blows. They dealt with early morning fog and nearly ran aground on Long Point, Lake Erie. But generally making good time, they reached the mouth of the Detroit River on August 10, where they picked up Tonty. Hennepin was quite impressed with the countryside along the Detroit River:

> The Country between those two Lakes is very well situated and the Soil very fertile. The Banks of the Streight are vast Meadows, and the Prospect is terminated with some Hills covered with Vineyards, Trees bearing good Fruit, Groves and Forests, so well dispos'd, that one would think Nature alone could not have made, without the Help of Art, so charming a Prospect. The Country is stocked with Stags, Wild Goats, and Bears, which are good for Food, and not fierce as in other Countries; some think they are better than our Pork. Turkey-Cocks and Swans are there also very common; and our Men brought other Beasts and Birds, whose Names are unknown to us, but they are extraordinary relishing. The Forests are chiefly made up of Walnut-trees, Chestnut-trees, Plum-trees and Pear-trees, loaded with their own Fruit and Vines. There is also abundance of Timber fit for Building; so that those who shall be so happy as to inhabit that Noble Country, cannot but remember with Gratitude those who discover'd the way, by venturing to sail upon an unknown Lake for above one hundred Leagues. That charming Streight lies between 40 and 41 Degrees of Northern Latitude.

Getting through Lake St. Clair presented problems. They were forced to sound continuously because of the ever-present shallows and finally found a channel without any shoals, and made their way upstream through the currents to the entrance into Lake Huron. Hennepin felt that the flow here was as violent as that of the Niagara River. Finally, they ordered twelve men ashore who hauled the ship safely into Lake Huron on August 23. They experienced a storm crossing Saginaw Bay but lay becalmed in Thunder Bay. Later they encountered a "furious gale," which caused La Salle to fear for the lives of his crew and passengers. Luc, the pilot, raged and swore at La Salle for bringing him to "a nasty freshwater lake to die, whereas he had lived long and happy navigating the ocean."

On August 27, they anchored off St. Ignace where they found a village of Huron Natives, a few of the Ottawa tribe, plus some French fur traders, coureur de bois and some Jesuit missionaries. Here La Salle was told that his 15-man advance party, sent ahead the previous year to collect furs, had deserted, but could be found some thirty leagues to the north at present-day Sault Ste. Marie. He sent Tonty north to arrest them and bring them back. After waiting for six days for him to return, La Salle headed for Green Bay in the *Griffon*.

La Salle was infuriated, frustrated and worried by the possibility that perhaps the entire advance party had deserted. Financial failure in this adventure could cost him everything, for his creditors were hounding him without mercy and had even taken possession of his estate at Fort Frontenac. He had intended to place Tonty in charge of the *Griffon* for the return journey to Niagara, but with this snap decision to send him after the deserters, La Salle was left only with his unreliable pilot, Luc, for that responsibility. It appears that La Salle's one rash decision (sending Tonty after the deserters) may have been the single act, more than any other, that was the direct cause of the failure of his expedition.

They left St. Ignace on September 2, and sailed down the Lake of the Illinois (now Lake Michigan) to an island just at the mouth of "the Bay of the Puans." The island was occupied by Potawatomi First Nation. La Salle was pleasantly surprised to find some of his advance party here, along with a large stock of furs that they had obtained in trade.

There is an unsolved mystery surrounding the rendezvous island. Hennepin writes that it was "forty leagues from Missillimac" and also refers to it as the island of the Potawatomi at the entrance to La Grande Baie," now known as Green Bay in Wisconsin. Various writers have attempted to prove the site to be Summer Island, Rock Island or Washington Island, but the controversy continues. The forty leagues described by Hennepin, when translated into today's measurements (one league equals 2.7 miles), and considering Hennepin's means of measurement, that is to say, the guess of a non-mariner, could establish the location anywhere among the islands strung out between the peninsula of Door County, Wisconsin, and Garden Island, Michigan.

Hennepin offers another clue, "Our Ship was riding in the Bay about thirty Paces from the furthermost Point of the Land, in a pretty good Anchorage, where we rode safely, not withstanding a violent Storm which lasted four Days." Where could La Salle have anchored safely for four or five days?

There are four locations worthy of consideration: 1) The harbour on the north coast of Summer Island, well protected from all but northeast winds and having good anchorage in 8 to 26 feet on today's charts; 2) The open roadstead south of Rock Island, protected from the southwest around west to north, but wide open from the northeast, east and southeast, and having extensive rocky shoals. Today's charts show a rocky bottom, seven to twenty-four feet in depth; 3) The west side of the sandy spit off Rock Island is better, but this location offers poor protection; 4) Detroit Harbour on Washington Island, protected on all sides and having narrow entrances but only seven to ten feet deep. We do not know the depth in 1679, but it is unlikely La Salle anchored in here, as today the small harbour is in use only as a result of having been dredged.

It appears certain that La Salle had instructed the men he sent ahead to rendezvous with the *Griffon* at a specific location, but Hennepin did not spell out any details for us, only stating that the ship rode out a four-day storm there. He later describes the island as four leagues north of the mainland of Door Peninsula. This sounds more like Rock Island than either of the others. Detroit Harbour is only about two leagues hence. Summer Island is nearer by ten leagues

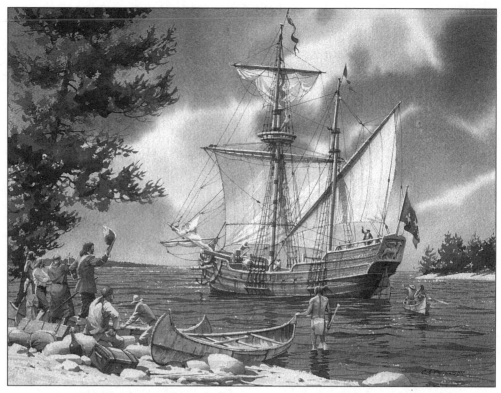

La Salle waves "Bon Voyage" to Luc and his men aboard the Griffon *as they head back to the Niagara River. He never saw them or the* Griffon *again. Charles L. Peterson, artist, 1978.*

from the mainland. Undoubtedly, all of these islands were used by the Native Peoples of the period. Native villages were reported on Washington, Rock and on Summer islands. The Jesuit priest, Pierre François-Xavier de Charlevoix[1] in 1721, describes a Potawatomi village on "one of the smallest of these islands." One would have expected La Salle to provide better protection for his *Griffon* than was obtainable at Rock or Summer, but it seems he showed considerable irresponsibility in the matter of her safety. Having sailed these waters in my own boat, which is about half the size of the *Griffon*, I would not want to anchor overnight at Summer, least of all at Rock, whereas Detroit is well protected in the worst of weather. I have experienced a lengthy and violent storm in these waters, and cannot see a small vessel riding safely in any but Detroit Harbour. Heavy rollers would have made the south coast of Rock and the north coast of Summer untenable; neither could be described as a "pretty good anchorage" under such circumstances. The determination of "the" island is of interest to historians and scholars only. For the purpose of the *Griffon* story it is really of little consequence.

The trade goods, ship-building tools and supplies were off-loaded for further transporting by canoe to Crèvecoeur. The furs were put on board, but, as noted, La Salle made the fatal mistake of sending the *Griffon* back to Niagara with Luc the pilot in charge and with only a skeleton crew of five men.

Hennepin's narrative continues with the comment on La Salle's feelings at having to do this:

> He was filled with forebodings for the safety of his vessel. Without asking anybody's Advice resolv'd to send back his Ship to Niagara with Furrs and Skins to discharge his Debts; our Pilot and five men were therefore sent back. They sailed the 18th of September with a Westerly Wind, and fir'd a gun to take their leave. Tho' the Wind was favourable, it was never known what Course they steer'd, nor how they perish'd; for after all the Enquiries we have been able to make, we could never learn any thing else but the following Particulars.
>
> The Ship came to an Anchor to the North of the Lake of the Illinois, where she was seen by some Savages, who told us that they advised our Men to sail along the Coast, and not towards the middle of the Lake, because of the Sands that make the Navigation dangerous when there is any high wind. Our Pilot, as I said before, was dissatisfy'd, and would steer as he pleas'd without hearkening to the Advice of the Savages, who generally speaking, have more Sense than the Europeans think at first; but the Ship was hardly a League from the Coast, when it was toss'd up in a violent Storm in such a manner, that

our Men were never heard of since; and it is suppos'd that the Ship struck upon a Sand, and was there bury'd. This was a great loss for M. la Salle and other Adventurers; for that Ship, with its Cargo, cost above sixty thousand Livres.

This is certainly not the first time that "local knowledge" has been ignored, nor the last. She was never heard from again!

No one knows for sure the fate of the *Griffon*. The cards were stacked against her from the beginning. The mystery of her final resting place may never be solved and her location is still being actively debated today. She headed out into Lake Michigan on that fateful September day and simply disappeared. Many theories have been brought forward in the literature in the intervening years. Many a "wreck of the *Griffon*" has been discovered, though all but one has been proven to be in error. No irrefutable evidence has been produced, such as Louis d'Or coins minted earlier than 1679, or one of her cannon with a fleur-de-lys embossed into it, nor any other hard evidence.

The find that received the most attention was in a cove on Russell Island, off Tobermory. The remains of an ancient vessel of about the right size was found by Orie Vail, a local fisherman.[2] The wreck was salvaged in the 1950s with much publicity. C.H.J. Snider wrote several articles about the find for historic publications, as did Rowley Murphy[3] an amateur historian and friend of Snider. Harrison John MacLean, another amateur historian wrote a book about the find,[4] but this has all been debunked. The Research Division of the National Historic Parks and Sites Branch of Parks Canada investigated the find in 1975 and concluded that the wreck was probably a gunboat of the type used at nearby Penetanguishene, a naval station established about the end of the War of 1812.

The one remaining find, which has neither been proven nor disproven, was in the Mississagi Passage at the western end of Manitoulin Island. This find was first reported around 1890. According to Native legend, the wreck had been there for a "hundred years" before that. Some articles and human skeletons were found nearby that could have been connected to the *Griffon*, but no irrefutable proof was found. It is reported that one human jaw bone, of enormous size, purportedly being that of Luc the Dane, was found by John Holdsworth, assistant lightkeeper for the Missisagi Light, and one of the locals. Accompanied by his supervisor William Cullis, while the two of them were out searching for a suitable tree from which to cut a new sailboat mast, Holdsworth happened upon a cave with a small collection of strange antiquities. Unfortunately, few artifacts remain and the wreck has been much plundered over the years, or washed off into deep water many years ago.

Various theories have been expressed that Luc scuttled the *Griffon* and transported the furs overland to sell them at his own profit, or that he was taken prisoner by the Natives who, in turn, sold the furs in Montreal. There is little on which to base this conjecture although it seemed that La Salle may have believed it himself.

There was one other possibility; since the storm arose so soon after the *Griffon's* departure and was both severe and lengthy, it is quite possible that she was lost between Green Bay and the Straits of Mackinac. Perhaps she foundered on one of the numerous shoals off the north shore of Lake Michigan. Sometime later, La Salle learned from the mission station at St. Ignace that a wooden "button" (cap) from the top of the *Griffon's* ensign staff, a hatch cover, two pairs of breeks and a pack of mouldy beaver skins had been cast up on the west side of Mackinac Island. These could have floated away from a vessel shipwrecked to the westward, but they give little indication of where the vessel went down. She could have been lost almost anywhere along the northern shore of Lake Michigan, along the Manitoulin shores or along the Bruce Peninsula.

One theory that has some merit is that she foundered somewhere between her point of departure and Mackinac Island. This could explain the finds on the western tip of Mackinac. And it is possible that the wreckage, with crew on board, then drifted to the Mississagi Channel. There it could have been tossed up on the rocky shore of Manitoulin Island, where the skeletons and other articles were found.

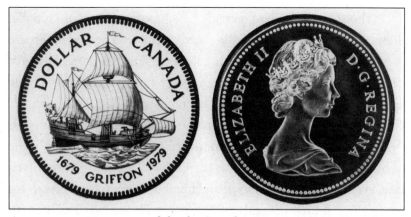

A commemorative coin struck by the Canadian Mint in 1979, recognizing the 300th anniversary of the Griffon. Courtesy of the Canadian Mint, Ottawa.

This is well within the limits of possibility and could explain the two finds, some miles apart. Incidentally, parts of the Manitoulin wreck were submitted to the National Academy of Arts and Trades in Paris, France, in 1931. The report indicates the metal parts were of a type manufactured in France prior to 1800. They might have been part of the *Griffon* or of some other vessel built before 1800 that used materials acquired from France. Furthermore, this wreck had used lead for caulking, a custom not used before or after in North America but a practice that was common in parts of Europe in the 1600s.

The fate of the *Griffon* continues to be debated even today. In the summer of 2006, an article appeared in the Detroit *Free Press* on August 24, 2006, mentioning the ill-fated ship once again. A sports diver, Steve Libert, believes he may have found the wreck of the *Griffon* in 100 feet of water in northeast Lake Michigan. Carbon-dating tests on small samples of wood from this wreckage indicate that it dates back to around the late 1670s, the time of the *Griffon*. Several groups, including the Center for Maritime and Underwater Resource Management at St. Johns, Michigan, are assisting Libert's company, the Great Lakes Exploration Group, with further studies. The immediate problem seems to be a territorial complication. The State of Michigan is claiming jurisdiction over the wreckage and the matter is not yet resolved.[5] Feel free to draw your own conclusions. It is unlikely the mystery will ever be definitively solved!

The story of the *Griffon* ends here, but the stories of La Salle, Tonty, Hennepin and of La Salle's men continue. These accounts are available in public libraries, with a little digging. They make absorbing reading of hardship, massacre, assassination and the indomitable spirit of La Salle. La Salle walked overland from Crèvecoeur, on the Illinois River, to Fort Frontenac in the dead of winter, and returned by canoe to continue his explorations only to be assassinated by some of his own party on the shores of the Gulf of Mexico. Tonty outlived him, ever resourceful, ever loyal and humble, a famous explorer in his own right, but little remembered in history. He is a figure well worth reading about.

How do we now commemorate this famous expedition? There is a bronze plaque erected at Tobermory by the Great Lakes Cruising Club. Four tiny islands off the north shore of the North Channel in Lake Huron (in an area that it is unlikely these early explorers ever saw) are named: Talon Rock, La Salle Island, Tonty Island and Hennepin Island. In 1979, three hundred years after the loss, the Canadian Government struck a silver commemorative dollar with an artist's rendition of the *Griffon* on one side. There are also communities bearing the name La Salle in Colorado, Illinois, Ontario and Quebec, plus a community called Hennepin that can be found in Oklahoma.

CHAPTER 4

The French Era Ends

FOLLOWING THE HIGH-PROFILE AND INTRIGUING story of the *Griffon* with all its mysteries, the next hundred or so years on the Great Lakes did not contain anything so exciting even though events are very well documented. We are not concerned here with political, military, nor economic history, except as it may impinge on our interest in sail. However, the events such as the Seven Years War, the uprising led by Pontiac, the Revolutionary War and the preparations for the War of 1812 must be touched upon to provide the historical context for our story, though not as fully as an historian might do.

In 1685, La Barre, Frontenac's successor, had a barque built at Cataraqui, which was named *Le General*. Little is known of her, other than she plied Lake Ontario for several years and made three trips to Niagara in 1688. There is some doubt as to whether *Le General* was a new vessel or one of La Salle's four earlier ships that had been rebuilt. Later, a fleet of flat-bottomed transports were added. Although these were hardly sailing ships, they did carry four-cornered lugsails. In 1687, the French launched a major attack against the Iroquois using the ships already mentioned and 198 such transports.

The French abandoned Fort Frontenac in 1688, and burned two of their ships at that time to prevent others from using them. No record has been found of what happened to the third, though in 1694, when the French re-occupied the fort, they raised one vessel from the harbour bottom, rebuilt her and put her into service.

The next shipbuilding, of which any record exists, was in 1726 when two schooners were built at Fort Frontenac by Intendant Bégin. In 1743 and 1745, Chevalier de Chalet added two more, the *St. Charles* and the *St. François*. Both were about 50 tons burthen. In 1734, Louis Denis, Sieur de la Ronde was sent by the governor of New France, to explore and report on the copper deposits at Chequamegon in 1727. He built a barque at Point aux Pins on Lake Superior for the copper mines at Chaguamagon, now part of Wisconsin. She was the second sailing vessel on the Upper Lakes and the first vessel to be described as sloop-rigged. It is not known what happened to her. The next mention of sail on Lake Superior concerns the English trader, Alexander Henry, in 1770. He could possibly have been using the same vessel, though this is unlikely.

About this time the "goelette" (an early version of the schooner) and the schooner started to come into use on the lakes but there are not sufficient records of early ships to indicate the exact date of their arrival.

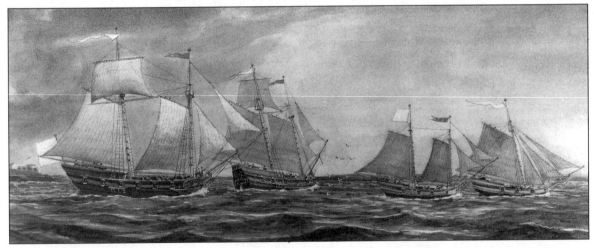

The French fleet of 1757 as depicted by Captain Pierre Bouchard de la Broquerie. The ships are (from left to right) La Marquise de Vaudreuil, La Hurault, La Louise *and* Le Victor. Courtesy of TRL-T15213.

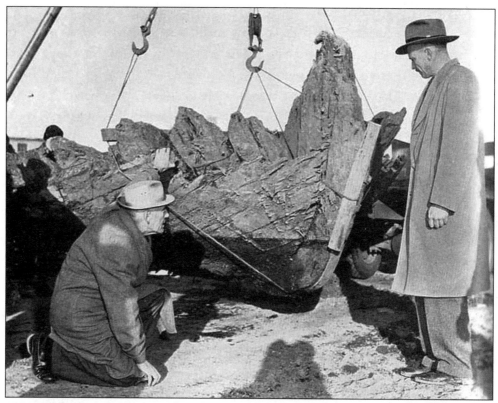

The director of the Old Fort Henry Museum, Ronald I. Way (right) and C.H.J. Snider examine the prow brought up from the foundation excavations at the National Defence College, Kingston, Ontario, December 16, 1953. After long study, the fragment was tentatively identified as the forefoot of the French man-of-war schooner La Hurault, *which had been launched at almost that identical spot some 200 years before, and burned and sank there after a battle in 1758. Taken from C.H.J. Snider,* Tarry Breeks and Velvet Garters, *1958.*

Several vessels were built at Cataraqui (now known as Kingston, Ontario) in the period from 1743 to 1756:

> *Le Victor:* 1749, 40-ton, schooner rig but later
> changed to sloop, 4 guns.
> *La Louise* (or *Lionne*): 1750, 50-ton schooner, 6
> guns.
> *La Hurault:* 1755, 90-ton schooner, 14 guns.
> *La Marquise de Vaudreuil:* 1756, 120-ton schooner,
> 20 guns.

Three lateen-rigged gunboats, names unknown, and two schooners, one large and one small, were built at Niagara but were not launched before they were captured by the British in July 1759. Records indicate that four vessels were built by the French at Navy Island, but it has not been possible to discover their names nor what happened to them. However, in 1836, Richard Bonnycastle, an officer in His Majesty's forces at Kingston and Toronto, mentioned a vessel raised from the waters and put on exhibition at Kingston. But to date, no connection has been determined.

In 1953, excavators on the site of the National Defence College at Kingston uncovered the remains of four wooden vessels. The forefoot of one hull was rather well preserved. It was believed to be the schooner, *La Hurault*, though this was not proven absolutely. In all, the French ignored their vulnerability on Lake Ontario. They had controlled the lakes unmolested up to now and did not foresee the need for more ships to protect their position until it was too late.

Governor William Shirley of Massachusetts receives credit for starting British shipbuilding on the lakes in order to compete with the French fur trade, and to protect the British settlements from the French and their Indian allies. He ordered the building of several ships of war at Choueguen (now Oswego, New York) in 1754 and brought in artificers from New York and Boston. Initially, all of the supplies and equipment were carried overland from the same towns, in spite of almost constant attacks and harassment by both the French and the Natives. The route, at first, was through the wilderness, up the Hudson, over the Mohawk trail, Lake Oneida and Carrying Place to the post at Oswego. Later, a stores depot was established at Schenectady, the upper navigable limit of the Hudson River.

In spite of horrendous difficulties, when Shirley arrived at Oswego in July of 1755, the vessels were almost ready for launching. Records indicate that these first British vessels on the lakes were essentially similar to those of the British navy in other areas. In fact, they were probably built to the designs of Sir J. Acworth, surveyor general of the Royal Navy.

They were pretty little craft, the *Ontario* and the *Oswego*, sister ships, each single-masted, gaff-rigged, fore-and-aft sloops. They were some 43 feet between perpendiculars with a 15-foot beam, taking some seven-foot draft when loaded. They would be of about 100 tons gross and were armed with five guns, 8- and 12-pounders, and at least one swivel cannon per side. Launched in 1755, they were the first vessels to enter ship-to-ship combat on the Great Lakes. Building continued in spite of frequent attacks by marauding Natives who continued to be loyal to the French.

Two schooners, the *George* and the *Vigilant*, soon followed down the ways. Their dimensions are unknown, but they were probably not larger than the earlier sloops, for they could be moved by sweeps (oars) if becalmed. They were armed the same as the *Ontario* and *Oswego*. Altogether eleven ships were built between the years 1755 and 1759. One hundred whaleboats, pinnaces and galleys were added to the small fleet, all in readiness for an assault on Fort Frontenac and Niagara. The vessels were manned by mariners from the coast, merchant sailors, whalers, naval crew and even deserters from British ships, and were officered by British Naval officers. This was an amazing feat of shipbuilding in the wilderness. Acquiring supplies created great problems, whether these were items needed for the construction, food and provisions for the men building the boats or items needed for the garrison at the fort.

The ships patrolled for three weeks in June 1756 without seeing any French sail until, on June 27, they were engaged by four French ships. After being fired on by the French, the British ships bore away, but one small British schooner, name unknown, was captured. The French ships headed back to port as neither side considered they should risk any additional loss.

On July 3 two more ships were launched by the British, the brig *London* and the sloop *Mohawk*, 172 tons. Later in the month the snow, *Halifax*, went down the ways. Additional whaleboats and other small boats continued to be added to the fleet. Although they cruised the lake for several weeks without incident, they were all in Oswego when Louis Joseph, Marquis de Montcalm[1] attacked overland from his base at Cataraqui on August 14, 1756, and took them by surprise.

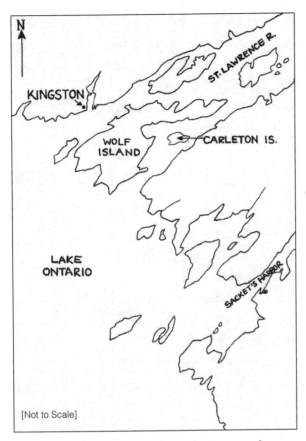

Sketch map of the eastern end of Lake Ontario, showing Sacket's Harbor and Kingston. Map by Heidi Hoffman.

Skipping over all the details of mismanagement and of incompetence and supply troubles, it is noted that the entire enterprise, fort, munitions and ships, were surrendered to the French. Fort Ontario at Oswego was destroyed, though most of the armaments and supplies were taken, along with all the vessels. The *Halifax* was renamed *Le Montcalm*, the *Ontario* became *L'Ontario*, the *Oswego, La Choueguine*, the *London, Le Jeorge* (or *L'Huron*), and the *Mohawk* became *Le Vigillent*.

Thus ended, for the moment, British attempts at naval and military power on Lake Ontario. The French had added six new ships to their fleet, courtesy of the British, whereas the latter had a complement of zero. The most outstanding accomplishment of this two-year period (1755-56) was the extent of shipbuilding that was achieved, starting from scratch, in a locale (Oswego), which, up to that time, had been little more than a small Indian settlement.

Both British and French soon embarked on a shipbuilding race, but up until 1760 the vessels saw little action and were employed primarily for transportation and dispatch. Some writers have claimed that the French built the *Montcalm* and the *Huron* at Fort Frontenac in 1756, but it appears certain that the new ships added to the French fleet were indeed the captured British vessels. However, several gunboats fitted with lugsails and sweeps were constructed there.

In 1758, Lieutenant-Colonel John Broadstreet was directed to raise a force of sailors, soldiers and landsmen in New England and to raid Fort Frontenac. By August 22, they had built sufficient whale-boats and bateaux. With their allies, the Oneida First Nation, they coasted along the south shore, crossed the lake at night and avoided detection until they had taken position only 200 yards from the fort. Broadstreet called on the French to surrender, which they did, and Fort Frontenac fell without a shot being fired. The British also captured nine French ships and all but two were burned. All the stores that could be carried were put into the *Montcalm*[2] and taken back to Oswego.

The British now occupied both Oswego and Fort Frontenac, and took Niagara in the summer of 1759. Later that year, they launched two schooners, the *Johnson* and the *Murray* at Niagara, and, later still, they launched the snow *Onondaga*. The following year they added the snow *Mississaga* at Oswego and the snow *Mohawk* at Niagara.

The French introduced two new vessels to Lake Ontario though they were built at L'Anse à la Construction in the lee of Pointe au Baril, now Maitland, Ontario, located in eastern Ontario along the shore of the St. Lawrence River. On April 9, 1759, a ship-rigged corvette, *L'Iroquoise*, was launched and on the 12th of the month, a barque, *L'Outaouaise*. The latter was of the same general size and ton-nage as the *Montcalm*, which had been captured by Broadstreet whereas the *L'Iroquoise* was slightly smaller. During the summer they put in good service carrying supplies to Fort Niagara but returned to the St. Lawrence to winter. Early in 1760, they were back on Lake Ontario but, as there was no port under French control that they could put in to, they returned to the St. Lawrence once again.

L'Iroquoise ran aground in the St. Lawrence River on August 13, and was no longer fit for service. She went down to Île Royale where she was later captured by the English on August 18 and sunk. The British, with a large flotilla of small boats, came up the St. Lawrence and, near present-day Brockville, did battle with the *L'Outaouaise*. The sad encounter was not unlike a pack of wolves attacking a large stag. Unfortunately for the French, the big ship was becalmed and thus without hope for escape. At noon, she lowered her fleur-de-lys and surrendered. The British took her over, and renamed her the

Williamson. She assisted them in the attack on Fort Levis, Île Royale, where the last shot in the "French-English" war was fired. She served on Lake Ontario until she was lost in a storm in November 1761.

In the 1990s, two divers, Michael Hughes and Dennis McCarthy, identified a wreck as the *L'Iroquoise*. She sits on the bottom in the narrows near the International Bridge, on what is known as Niagara Shoal, between the mainland and Wellesley Island in the St. Lawrence River, where today the bridge crosses from Ontario to New York State. The *Mohawk* and the *Onondaga* were lost in 1764, but the details are not known.

This action ended French naval power on Lake Ontario and in the St. Lawrence, however, they still had outposts at Detroit and Mackinac. On September 12, 1760, the famous Roger's Rangers, an independent company of light infantry attached to the British army, set out from Montreal in fifteen small whaleboats. Their objective was to capture Detroit. They travelled up the rapids of the St. Lawrence, along the north shore of Lake Ontario, portaged around Niagara and continued the length of Lake Erie. At the mouth of the Detroit River they met Pontiac,[3] chief of the Ottawa, who had been loyal to the French. At the time he displayed a "peaceful attitude," but later would lead an Indian uprising against the encroachment of the British on Native lands. On November 12, 1760, the Rangers captured the French fort at Detroit. Fort Mackinac, in the Straits of Mackinac, was turned over to the British the following year.

The Great Lakes saw no action for the next period as attention shifted to the American War of Independence. From 1775 to 1777 it was a war between Great Britain and the thirteen British colonies that had declared their independence as the United States of America in 1776.[4] The revolution was settled by the 2nd Treaty of Paris in 1783 when the British representatives were hopelessly out-manoeuvred at the negotiating table. They showed a great deal of ignorance of both the geography and the potential of the remaining colonies, that is to say, in Canada, and of Britain's own strength in the colonial domain. The British negotiators conceded much and ceded a great deal of land that had been garnered up over a century

of effort. They did get a promise, of sorts, from the American negotiators to restore confiscated property and make restitution to the
Loyalists and to the citizens of Britain who had invested in the
Thirteen Colonies. The Americans also promised that there would
be no more confiscation of property.

Neither of these promises was kept. Britain herself recompensed
many Loyalists and, in fact, spent between 30 and 40 million dollars,
but a great many of these colonists affected by the war received very
little or nothing. They suffered great hardship, both physical and
financial. Britain tried to force payment from the Americans and
refused to give up its posts along the new international boundary,
(Oswego, Detroit, Michillimackinac, etc.) and by doing so, she
retained control of the contiguous land and the fur trade that took
place across these territories.

By a second treaty, the Treaty of Amity (or better known as Jay's
Treaty) in 1794, Britain agreed to give up these posts and the
Americans agreed to pay their obligations. The posts were relin-
quished, however, the obligations were never paid.

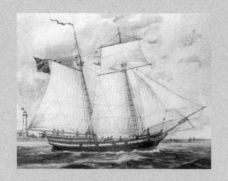

PART TWO

Events From 1760
Until After the War of 1812

"Let us remember famous men and our fathers who begat us."

"They built great ships and sailed them" sounds most brave
Whatever arts we have or fail to have,
I touch my country's mind. I come to grips
With half her purpose, thinking of these ships.
– John Masefield

The Toronto, C.H.J. *Snider, artist.* Courtesy of the Toronto Reference Library
(TRL) T15210.

CHAPTER 5

Between the Wars

THE RECORDS OF SHIPS IN THESE EARLY YEARS are very difficult to sort out. The names of vessels were often changed. This usually happened when a vessel switched ownership, or, of course, if she were captured in times of war and moved into the fleet of the victor. Also, when a ship was sunk, wrecked or even grew too old to be of further use and was retired, a new one frequently acquired the same name. It was not uncommon for two vessels to carry the same name at one time. The most renowned writers were apt to be confused at times by these circumstances and they often disagreed. Anyone who wishes to dig deeper into the pedigrees of the commercial ships of the period is referred to the book by George Cuthbertson, and the series of books which make up the *American Lake Series*, plus *Our Inland Seas* by J.C. Mills.[1] The history books written in the late 20th century are generally excellent at recounting the details of military events in this period. A superb list of British naval vessels was prepared by K.R. Macpherson and published in *Ontario History*.[2] Be forewarned that there is plenty of disagreement among historians, but these titles make a good starting point. However, in this context, these events are only touched upon as they concern my subject and mandate.

When the British captured Fort Niagara in 1759, they also won two partially built schooners and the material for finishing them. The two ships were completed and launched in September of that year, the *Johnson* and the *Murray*. In 1760, a snow was launched at Niagara, the *Onandaga*, and another snow, the *Misissaga*, launched at Oswego. This was one way to augment the British fleet. Cuthbertson describes a snow as, "vessels of three masts square rigged on the fore and main masts and lateen rigged on the mizzen."

Captain Joshua Loring RN was put in charge of the naval forces on the lakes. He had been involved in building the British ship at Oswego, served on Lake Champlain in 1759 and on the St. Lawrence River in 1760. Although badly wounded in the attack on Fort Levis, he remained in charge of the vessels on the Upper Lakes until 1765. The activity at Navy Island and the forays during the Pontiac uprising were part of his career. His early efforts formed the base upon which the Provincial Marine was built.[3]

At this time traders, settlers, hunters and trappers from the colonies to the south and from Montreal and Quebec, invaded the lakes to take advantage of the fur trade that the French had been forced to abandon. The British needed some way to protect and service the area, and to transport men and supplies from Niagara westward, hence they started to use the old French shipyard on Navy Island. This site is in the Niagara River, some three miles above the lip of the Falls (the French called it "Île de la Marina"). In 1762, they built two ships, the *Huron* and the *Michigan*. While some authors give these vessels other names, Cuthbertson's research in *Freshwater* seems indisputable. These ships were of some 80-tons displacement, 60 feet long, 14 feet wide, schooner-rigged and armed with three four-pounders on each side. Each carried two swivel-mounted guns at the bows. They saw some exciting action in the Detroit River during the Pontiac uprising and were present during the attack on Fort Mackinac on June 2, 1763.[4] The *Michigan* was shipwrecked at Point Albino, along the south shore of Lake Erie between present-day Buffalo and Erie, Pennsylvania, on August 28, 1763. There is no information on the fate of the *Huron*. Two additional schooners were built on Navy Island in 1764 for service on the Upper Lakes, the *Royal Charlotte* and the *Victory*. Shipbuilding ceased here in 1764 until after the War of 1812, when the *Tecumseth* and the *Newash* were built and added to the fleet in 1815. Actually, they were completed at a site across a narrow part of the Niagara River at Chippawa.

In 1777, England proclaimed that the Provincial Marine was to control all shipping on the Great Lakes. Private ownership of ships was prohibited until 1788. Arms, supplies, merchandise and passengers were to be carried in none but the King's ships, however, the law was not followed to the letter. In fact, the authorities appear, at times, to have preferred the freedom to use privately-owned commercial ships. The yards at Oswego and at Kingston were idle, but shipbuilding continued at Oswegatchie (present-day Ogdensburg, New York), Carleton Island and Detroit. In 1790, a small sloop, the *Good Intent*, was built near Kingston. She was the first private vessel under the new regulations. In 1776, shipbuilding had been started at a yard on Carleton Island in the St. Lawrence River and two ships, the *Duke of Kent*, a schooner, and the *Caldwell*, a cutter, were built. These two vessels were added to the fleet of the Provincial Marine.

In 1778, Captain John Schank, who had been part of the Royal Navy along the Atlantic coast of America before the War of Independence, was brought up to Canada following the hostilities as he was loyal to the King. He is given credit with building up the British fleet for the Lake Champlain campaign during the War of 1812. He later became "Admiral of the Blue."[5] John Coleman, the master shipwright, who was trained in Royal Navy yards in England, had also been employed in the shipyards at Quebec. Together, Schank and Coleman built many whaleboats,[6] and three 60-foot gunships for the raid on the American shipyards at Oswego, which took place later that same year.

On May 10, 1780, the *Ontario* was launched at Carleton Island. She was a snow, 80 feet on deck and of 220 tons. She immediately went into service carrying troops, stores, merchandise, raiding parties and passengers. Captain James Andrews was in command. The next year, the *Mohawk* and the *Limnade* were launched there. The *Ontario*, on passage from Niagara to Carleton Island on October 31, 1780, was struck by the tail end of a hurricane and was lost. She was last seen from the north shore but on the next day, wreckage was found on the opposite shore, and bodies were recovered there the following spring. The same hurricane destroyed hundreds of vessels among the Caribbean islands, in Bermuda and in New England before hitting the Great Lakes. All hands on board were lost, the estimates ranging from as low as 40 to as high as 120 persons. The wreck of the *Ontario* was located in August 1995, by divers from Olcott, New York. An excellent book about the vessel and the yard at Carleton Island was written by Arthur Britton Smith, under the title, *Legend of the Lake: The 22-gun Brig-sloop, Ontario.*[7]

It is likely that Schank's shipyards on Lake Champlain and at Carleton Island were responsible for the training of local shipwrights who later continued to ply their trade all around the lower lakes. The yards were well-known in their time. The *General Haldimand*, built at Oswegatchie in 1771, sank at her moorings in Schank's Harbour, Carleton Island, in November 1787. However, commercial ships seem to have been built in just about every creek or harbour that had room for them to float and had a supply of timber nearby.

Hatcher in his 1945 book, *Lake Erie*, writes:

With little capital a man could build his sailing vessel at modest cost and to any size from a ten-ton sloop to a three-masted schooner. Its only fuel was the wind, and the wind was free. The captain-owner and his sons or his nephews, or the neighbour boys, could sail her down from Port Talbot to Buffalo with a cargo of lumber, or out of Huron with a few tons of grain, or up to Detroit with butter and wheat and

hardware. The first American vessel built on the
Upper Lakes was launched at Presque Isle in 1796.[8]

He also tells about vessels being built at Black Rock, on the
American side of the Niagara River, because Buffalo had no adequate
harbour. Unless by some miracle they were favoured by a ten-knot
wind from the east, they had to be towed up the river and into Lake
Erie. The towing service was known as the "horned breeze." From
"eight to fourteen yoke of oxen" were used to haul a ship.

As noted earlier, the *Limnade* (sister ship to the *Ontario*) was
launched in 1781. She was the first Great Lakes vessel to be ship-
rigged, that is to say, to have three masts, all square-rigged. *Limnade*
means "water nymph," but the ship was referred to at times as the
"*Lemonade*." She seems to have had a short, but rather peaceful life,
and was written off and sunk at Kingston after only ten years of
service.

In 1794, a small shipyard was started at Chatham, on the
Thames River. Because pine was not available to the builders, black
walnut was substituted for the timber. Six gunboats were to be built,
sawn to a thickness of half an inch. Two vessels were completed, but
the shipyard was closed in 1796 and a new one was created at
Amherstburg along the Detroit River.

In 1788, the British government altered the rules of the Provincial
Marine regarding the organizing of armed vessels on the Great Lakes
and permission was granted for privately owned vessels to engage in
commerce on the lakes. However, the size of the ship was limited to
90 tons burthen. Certainly, larger ones were built, but they were registered at 90 tons or less, a creative response to the limitations.

While the first sailing ship to appear in the Detroit River was,
of course, the *Griffon* (it had passed up the river on August 11, 1679),
by November of 1760 the British had taken Fort Detroit, and soon
after captured the French bases at Michillimackinac, Sault Ste. Marie
and St. Joseph (on St. Joseph Island about 20 miles downstream from
present-day Sault Ste. Marie, Ontario). From that point on, the
French retired from the lakes for all time.

Actually, in the 1760s, a British shipyard was in operation at Detroit at the water's edge at the foot of today's Woodward Avenue, and, later, another yard appeared on the River Rouge on the southerly side of Fort Street, near the site of present-day Woodmere Cemetery. For some time the British had been building their ships at Navy Island, but now the main activity shifted to Detroit. It appears obvious from old records that British ships were frequenting both Lake Michigan and Lake Huron regularly, for in 1767, Sir William Johnson,[9] in his report to the Board of Trade in London, urged the establishment of a fort in Green Bay (Wisconsin) stating, "It can receive all its supplies in the King's ships which go to Michillimackinac without additional expense."

In his 1963 article, K.R. Macpherson lists thirteen additional ships built by the British at Detroit for the Provincial Marine between 1772 and 1791. More detail on them will appear in connection with the War of 1812. One in particular, the *Nancy* (built in 1789), receives particular attention. In 1775, at Michillimackinac, a private trading vessel, the *Welcome*, was constructed for John Askin of Detroit, a fur trader, merchant and an official of Upper Canada.[10] She was a square-rigged sloop, 55 feet overall, with a 16-foot beam and a gross tonnage of 45. In 1779, she was purchased by the Provincial Marine to be used to supply the fort. She plied the lakes until 1781, when she was lost with all hands to an unknown grave.

Commercial shipbuilding continued at an ever-increasing pace. In 1792-93, the 50-ton top-sail schooner *Detroit* was built and launched at Detroit. She was purchased by the United States government and was armed, but was not taken into the navy. James Mills, in *Our Inland Seas*, writes that she was wrecked in 1797.

In 1796, the American Fur Company, of which John Jacob Astor[11] was principal shareholder, was established at Detroit and Michillimackinac, trading into the entire northwest on both sides of the border. Astor was to have a great influence on events on the lakes, not only in commerce but also through his pressuring the US government to declare war on the British in 1812 so that he might obtain mastery over the fur trade in the northwest for his own company.

The schooner *Washington* was built at Presque Isle (now Erie, Pennsylvania), some 80 tons in size, in 1797. She was purchased by British buyers, and, in the winter of 1797-98, taken on huge skids across the Niagara Portage Road to Lake Ontario where she was renamed the *Lady Washington*. However, another *Washington* appears in the returns (the record of the vessels and cargos at each port each year) at Detroit for 1800. Presumably, she too was built at Detroit.

Mention was made earlier of ships being built in any creek or harbour where there was a supply of good timber. In 1798, John Askin sent the shipwright, William Daly, up the Thames to Delaware to build a boat for him. It was to have a 28-foot keel, 10-foot beam and a 4-1/2 foot hold, "deep enough to stow two Rows of Barrels over each other." She was to be built of white oak and there was to be a small cabin with two berths and the quarterdeck was to be a foot higher than the main deck. It was to cost £110.00. F.C. Bald writes that she was named the *Surprise*, that she was built at the Pinery in the vicinity of the present-day City of London, and that she saw service for many years.[12] In those days, many of the sailing vessels that were based on Lakes Erie, Huron and Michigan went up the Thames to trade, for the area was the "bread-basket" for early settlers until grain started to be imported from Chicago. (As an aside, while I am undertaking the final revisions to this story, I am much aware of living on the north bank of the Thames River in London on a ridge of fine old oaks. It is not difficult to look at these trees, huge and mature, and see knees, ribs, futtocks and planks within their trunks and massive limbs, and to visualize their place within the complex, hand-tooled structures of the early sailing ships.)

After the British surrendered Detroit on July 11, 1796,[13] they proceeded to strengthen and build ships at Fort Malden, across the river from Detroit, near Amherstburg. Soon this shipyard was turning out both commercial and naval vessels. In fact, in 1794, a schooner had been extensively rebuilt here and named the *Ottawa*, but where she originally was built and what her name had been before the rebuilding is not recorded. William Bell, a Scottish immigrant, was signed on as master shipwright in charge of the yard here in 1799.

Here, too, were constructed many of the British ships that saw service in the War of 1812.

In 1800, the brig *Recovery* (150 tons) was launched at Point aux Pins on Lake Superior, to be followed by the schooner *Perseverance* (80 tons) in 1803. The Americans captured her in July 1814 and tried to float her down the rapids at Sault Ste. Marie where she was wrecked and then set on fire. Mills, in *Our Inland Seas*, writes that the *Recovery* survived the war, passed down the rapids and saw service in the lumber trade on Lake Erie. The *Mink* was also built at Point aux Pins for the North West Company. She went down the rapids during the war, was captured and burned by the Americans in 1814.

In March 1803, the American War Department directed Colonel Randolph Hamtramck to establish a fort at the mouth of the Chicago River. Captain John Whistler sailed with his family on the *Tracy* with a load of artillery and other supplies for founding Fort Dearborn. The *Tracy* had been built at Detroit in 1799 and was the first of many sailing vessels to reach Chicago. Around the same time, in the same shipyard at Detroit, the *Adams* was built. She was a 150-ton brig and became the first of the American navy vessels on the Upper Lakes. She served until captured by the British when Detroit fell. Renamed the *Detroit*, she was anchored under the guns of Fort Erie when Lieutenant Jesse D. Elliott USN attempted to recapture her on October 9, 1812. He did not succeed and the *Detroit* was battered by the guns of both sides and destroyed in the Niagara River.

In 1808, the first United States Navy vessel to appear on Lake Ontario, the brig *Oneida*, was launched at Oswego. The builders were Henry Eckford and Christian Berg. She was 243 tons, with 16 guns, and served extensively in the war that was about to erupt. She was still in service as a timber drogher in 1828.

Interestingly, the American War of Independence was hardly noticed on the Great Lakes. During the revolution, the British prohibited commerce between the two countries, but the forbiddance had little effect. Following the outcome of this war, vast waves of refugees entered Canada from the south, people who had been loyal to the Crown and were seeking a new life where they could continue their loyalty. Stripped of their land and much of their possessions, these migrants became known as the United Empire Loyalists. The arrival of the Loyalists peaked around 1780, and the ships of the Provincial Marine were kept busy transporting them across Lakes Ontario and Erie.

Over the period of early sailing vessels on the Great Lakes, reports show that many were lost early in their careers. At the time there were no aids to navigation and the few charts available were very incomplete. In 1803, construction of the first lighthouses on the lakes was commenced at Kingston, Niagara and York. Of necessity, the early navigator learned quickly the need for constant alertness and caution. If he was careless, his prospects for a long life were no better than that of his ship.

CHAPTER 6

Events Leading Up to the War of 1812

HISTORY BOOKS VARY GREATLY in their recounting of a particular event. What is written often depends on the viewpoint and patriotic affiliation of the writer. Reading the stories of a battle as written by authors from both sides, one may have a hard time correlating each description with the actual event. Apart from date and place, one sometimes gets the impression that entirely different battles are being narrated. And generally the winner writes the history.

Each writer feels called upon to embellish the bravery and competence of "our boys" against overwhelming odds, and to cast aspersions on the intelligence and courage, even antecedents, of "theirs." Unless an event portrays "our boys" to the best advantage, the entire incident may be dropped from the history book. In fact, some of the early works concerning the war were largely boldfaced propaganda, with the addition of a few doubtful facts. One must dig deeply into the on-the-spot reports of officers and administrators and the diaries of the men whose blood was being spilled, in order to try to get at the hard and reliable facts. It was often difficult to determine which side had the bigger ships and more guns, the better strategists and leaders, or whatever. Even then, one must learn to read between the lines, compare the reports from the front lines of each protagonist and then form one's own opinion.

It is pleasant to be an armchair general, or admiral, and point out, from this vantage point in history, the errors in policy, mistakes in strategy and the incompetence in administration, so obvious now, which the men in power or in the battlefield of the day did not see. Or, perhaps, they did not choose to see.

"I do not believe that history is a force that we are somehow agents of. I believe history is made up. Otherwise we wouldn't have 20 different histories of the same event. History is something that you create. I get all the details correct when I want to," says George Bowering in Simon Fraser University's *Comment.*

The present work is not intended to be a nationalistic history, but rather is concerned primarily with events on the waters of the Great Lakes. As noted, politics is addressed only from an incidental perspective. Perhaps, as author, I shall be forgiven for including certain material that relates to political events or points of view generally ignored by some historians. Now approaching 200 years later, and looking back on history from this distance, it seems pointless to try to prove anything. After all, the settlers, soldiers and sailors on both sides of the lakes were of essentially the same stock. They must have been matched evenly in skills and courage. The differences, if any, were to be found among the leaders, and more particularly in the politicians and administrators, who, sitting back in the relative peace of Washington and London, sent "our boys" off to a war that should never have happened.

Undoubtedly there would have been a difference in attitude of the participants on both sides. For one it was a war to gain more land, more furs and more wealth. For the other side it was a necessity to protect their land and homes from what was seen as an aggressive and greedy neighbour. US Speaker of the House Henry Clay[1] wrote in 1810, "The conquest of Canada is in your [the American people] power. I trust I shall not be deemed presumptuous when I state that I verily believe that the militia of Kentucky are alone competent to place Montreal and Upper Canada at your feet." In contrast, in 1812, General Isaac Brock,[2] the commander of the land forces of Canada at the outbreak of the war, wrote, "A country defended by Free Men, enthusiastically devoted to the cause of their King and Constitution, can never be conquered."[3] Later, with some disillusionment, his sentiments would be expressed quite differently.

The war itself was a farcical affair in many ways, one that wiser leaders could have prevented. Once it was declared, however, it was entered into seriously by both sides, with a few notable exceptions. A very brief background, merely to set the scene, is in order here. Great Britain had been fighting, off and on since 1793, against Napoleon, who, from my perspective, was the greatest dictator the world had ever known. At times this war had placed Britain, on the one side, against almost all the other countries in Europe. In such a prolonged life-and-death struggle, a great deal depended on control of the seas, both to prevent invasion of the British Isles and to keep critical supplies out of the hands of the French.

The British navy lost many sailors through desertion for a variety of reasons: involuntary impressments (where men were forced into service by the opposing side), low pay, long periods at sea, cruel living conditions and others concerns. Britain was, at times, unable to operate all her vessels completely due to the shortage of men. Hence, she reserved the right to stop and search other vessels on the high seas, and to remove any British seamen. This she did repeatedly and at times removed not only deserters, but seamen who had emigrated to the United States (perhaps legally, perhaps not) in previous years. Deserters were usually hanged and the others were impressed into naval service. Undoubtedly, in the dire need for men, some Americans were included among those taken, though it should be noted that many Americans voluntarily served in the British fleet and conditions were not always cruel and hard. Furthermore, a seaman of any country could obtain an American Certificate of Citizenship, or "Protection" on short notice in many American ports or even on board some American merchant vessels, making it difficult to determine citizenship.

In order to prevent other nations from supplying articles of war or comfort to the French, the British declared it to be their right to stop such traffic and enacted Orders-in-Council in an attempt to blockade American ports. The United States naturally took the stand of support for "free ships, free trade." They demanded freedom of the seas for both American ships and for US sailors.

No one knew actually how many Americans were impressed into the British navy. It would be impossible to determine now. There is no doubt that the figure was blown out of all reality by factions intent on stirring up the nation to war. Future president, James Monroe[4] claimed in 1812 that over 6,000 Americans had been impressed, but that report was shot full of holes by the General Court of Massachusetts. Fifty-one of the leading ship owners of Massachusetts, who had employed annually over 1,500 seamen for the preceding twelve years, could remember only 12 instances of American sailors being impressed from their vessels.

The New England states, those most affected by embargo and impressments, were overwhelmingly against the war. In the Congressional deciding ballot, New England stood nineteen states to one for peace. Maine continued to ship timber and other supplies to Britain in spite of the embargo decreed by Washington, in exchange for British goods she needed, and from which she could profit. Smuggling constituted big business for a time, with the connivance of both ship owners and the authorities on both sides. Fortunes were amassed by supplying the British Army during the Napoleonic War in the Iberian Peninsula. For the first six months of the war, every Atlantic port traded with England, under licence from the British blockading squadron.

Great Britain was not the only nation guilty of impressment. France, too, coerced American seamen into her navy and wrought havoc on US shipping. Even Monroe, in 1812, admitted that Napoleon had done more harm to American commerce than had the British navy.

President James Madison[5] continued his efforts for peace and seemed to be making some headway toward agreement with the belligerents. But, the American Congress of 1811 contained a group of young men from the South and West, led by Henry Clay and John

Calhoun,[6] who brought into it a new spirit. No longer were its deci-
sions to be dominated by the Fathers of the Revolution. The rising
generation now manifested its power. The young "War Hawks," as
they were called, felt that the days were over when it was necessary
for the United States to temporize, just to delay the inevitable. The
slogan "Free Trade and Sailor's Rights" was coined by men who rarely,
if ever, saw a ship or a sailor. It was devised by a sectional combination of Congress that had neither commerce nor shipping at heart,
but used the call to rally the populace for purely political purposes.
Such slogans did much to stir the feelings of an otherwise docile citizenry into action. It would be a good time to strike, for Britain was
otherwise engaged, and weakened by years of war. The United States
could count on some measure of assistance from France now that she,
too, had declared herself at war with Britain.

The War of 1812–1814 has been called "The Incredible War"
and "Mr. Madison's War" and "The Shipbuilder's War," but perhaps it
should also be called "John Jacob Astor's War." One undeniable reason
for going to war resulted from Astor's greed for more control of new
lands for his fur trade. When, by treaty in 1794, Britain gave up
Detroit and Missillimackinac, Astor concluded, "Now I will make my
fortune." He deliberately bent the fledgling government to his own
uses. He had a great influence with President Madison and persuaded
him to have forts built to protect his monopoly in the American fur
trade against British intruders. He wanted exclusive rights to trade in
lands that were loosely controlled by the United States, but, by treaty,
also in those lands in which trade was conducted by the Hudson's Bay
Company and the North West Company. He also owned trading posts
in what was indisputably British territory.

Bowing to political and economic pressures, President Madison
acceded. On June 18, 1812, Congress declared a state of war to exist
with England. Ironically, the British Parliament had revoked her
Orders-in-Council, which were the key causes for the declaration,
five days earlier, thus removing one of the principal bones of con-
tention between the two countries. Congress, in declaring war,
showed exactly where its real interests lay. The legislators voted down

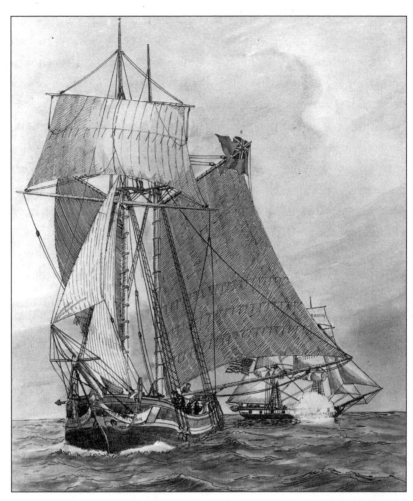

Capture of the Lord Nelson *by the American* Oneida *off Niagara on July 5, 1812,* C.H.J. Snider, *artist.* Courtesy of TRL, T15223.

a proposal to establish ships and to build up a navy to back up its demand for "Free Trade and Sailor's Rights." Instead, the members voted to increase the army from 10,000 to 35,000 soldiers, plus 50,000 volunteers, to attack Canada and push the frontiers to the north and to the west. These few facts are, of course, an over-simplification. However, they do serve to set the stage for the events that concern us on our inland waters.

A short war was expected by the Americans. They believed that, of course, the Canadians would welcome the invading forces with open arms. In fact, Lieutenant Melancthon Woolsey, a senior US officer on the Lakes, and commander of the brig, *Oneida*, operating out of Sacket's Harbor early in the season of 1812, called in at Kingston and York to recruit Canadians to join the US Navy. He met with no success. Woolsey may have been a good enough naval officer, but he was impulsive. In May, three weeks before war was declared by Congress, he had seized the British schooner *Lord Nelson*, operating on a packet freight run between Niagara and Kingston and carrying flour. The *Lord Nelson* was renamed the *Scourge* and armed with 12 guns, including a long 32-pound swivel cannon. Woolsey purchased other merchant schooners; *Elizabeth* (2 guns) as a transport; *Fair American* (82 tons, 2 guns); *Charles And Ann* (renamed *Governor Tomkins*) (6 guns); *Experiment* (renamed *Growler*) (53 tons, 2 to 6 guns); and the *Collector*, (renamed *Pert*) (3 guns). One writer claims Woolsey seized two other ships before war was declared, the *Niagara* and the *Ontario*.

As this narrative is concerned with neither the war on the high seas nor on land and as much has been written about these theatres and such treatises are readily available to the interested reader, the emphasis here continues on the Great Lakes. Since the aspirations of the United States were to expand north and west, the Great Lakes theatre was the most important of all. In June of 1812 neither side was in any respect equipped for war. Although the American plan was to sweep into Canada via Lake Champlain, across the Niagara-Lake Ontario frontier and the Detroit River-Lake Erie frontier, there were few ships available for that purpose.

The transportation of men, munitions and supplies was just as important for the success of the invading army as it was for the defence of Canada. The supply routes were, of necessity, by water, there being no roads worthy of the name. Control of the lakes was essential! All men and supplies for the defence of Upper Canada had to pass up the St. Lawrence (on foot or by sleigh in winter, by bateaux in summer) and through Kingston. Hence, Kingston was recognized as the linchpin of the campaign by both the aggressor and the defender.

There were, in fact, three different naval theatres on the lakes, Lake Champlain, Lake Ontario and the Upper Great Lakes. Each was completely cut off from the others, in that vessels could not be moved from one location to any other. Neither could the Royal Navy bring in any of its vast resources to support the war effort until later. These assets were well occupied elsewhere. As the war in Europe wound down, both armaments and men were gradually transferred to the Great Lakes.

Had the United States concentrated its efforts, early in the war, on cutting the British supply line at Montreal, or at Kingston, instead of devoting so much effort to other areas, the war, without doubt, would have ended much earlier, and with an entirely different outcome. From Kingston, the fastest supply route was by water to York or Niagara, overland to Fort Erie or the Grand River, then by water to Fort Malden or Mackinac. The alternative overland routes were slow, tedious and expensive (e.g. up the Ottawa, along Lake Nipissing and into Georgian Bay or from York overland to Lake Simcoe, then by portage to the Nottawasaga or Severn rivers and down to Georgian Bay). Such roads as there were became impassable in spring or following a heavy rain. Control of the lakes was definitely essential!

Canada had more settlers along the St. Lawrence and the lakes than did the United States but had no local industry suited to the making of munitions. England most certainly, but even Quebec, was a great distance away from the Great Lakes. On the United States side, supplies had to be brought from the seaboard cities via Albany, through the valley of the Mohawk. No canal was available, only very poor roads, augmented by transport on the Mohawk River, Lake Oneida and the Onondaga River to Oswego.

Pittsburgh is only 130 miles from Erie. In 1812 it had a population of 6,000. Among its industries, it numbered foundries, ropeworks, metal working shops, sawmills and much more. It was called the "Birmingham of America" and became an important supply base for the Erie shipyard. By 1812 there were good roads between Philadelphia and Pittsburgh. From Pittsburgh the Allegheny River and its tributary, the French Creek, provided water transport to within 15 miles from Erie. This last 15 miles had to be covered by road. However, much still had to come from more distant cities, New York and Washington, and there was the same difficult road transport problem that was faced by the other bases. Transport to Sacket's

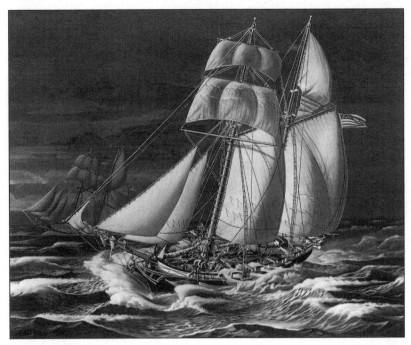

The Hamilton and the Scourge, *Duncan Macpherson, artist. On the night of August 8, 1813, a sudden squall hit both the* Hamilton *and the* Scourge *just off the mouth of the Niagara River. Both ships were overwhelmed and sank. The remains were found in 1973.* Courtesy of Dorothy Macpherson.

Harbor would be via Oswego. From here, the supplies could go by water to Sacket's or to Niagara, overland to Black Rock, then by water again to Erie or Detroit.

If one navy were the stronger, then the weaker side, by skilful harassment, could be content in keeping the sovereignty of the lake in dispute. As long as one side had to make allowances for the other, it could not be relied on to assist in transporting troops and munitions, attacking forts, or otherwise helping the land forces. Control of the lakes was indeed essential!

Earlier it was mentioned that the *Lord Nelson*, a small (50 ton) schooner, was taken before war was declared, and renamed the *Scourge*. She had been built at Newark by shipwright, Asa Stanard, for William Crooks, a Canadian, in 1811. At the time of capture, she was owned by William and James Crooks. James was a pioneer industrialist and prominent politician. After the war, he sued the United States for the value of the vessel and his family continued to pursue the claim. It was finally settled, but not until 116 years later, in 1930 for $23,644.38.

In October 1812, Captain Isaac Chauncey[7] of the United States Navy purchased the 76-ton schooner, *Diana*, and renamed her the *Hamilton*. Both the *Hamilton* and the *Scourge* were based at Sacket's Harbor and served until August 8, 1813, when both were overwhelmed in a squall and sunk near the mouth of the Niagara River with a loss of 53 lives. One of the survivors was Ned Meyers who, many years later, recounted the events of that night to the famous American novelist, James Fenimore Cooper. He, in turn, published the story in 1843, under the title *Ned Myers: or Life Before the Mast*. As Ned relates, "The flashes of lightning were incessant and nearly blinded me. Our decks seemed on fire, and yet I could see nothing. I heard no hail, no order, no call, but the schooner was filled with shrieks and cries of the men to leeward, who were lying jammed under the guns, shot-boxes, shot, and other heavy things that had gone down as the vessel fell over."[8] The story makes exciting reading, especially to one who has weathered white squalls and violent electrical storms out on Lake Ontario, in a much smaller boat, but with less serious consequences.

The well-preserved wrecks of the *Hamilton* and the *Scourge* were found in 1973 through the efforts of Dr. Daniel A. Nelson, a St. Catharines dentist, diver and amateur archaeologist, and Dr. A. Douglas Tushingham of the Royal Ontario Museum in Toronto. Many others helped in the investigation and documentation, including Jacques Cousteau[9] who arranged exploration of the wreck site and took extensive documentary photographs. An excellent story of the ships and their rediscovery has been written by Emily Cain and published in 1983 under the title, *Ghost Ships: Hamilton and Scourge*.

CHAPTER 7

Declaration of War

ON JUNE 18, 1812, the American Congress declared war.

At the outset, neither country was prepared. The Americans had bases at Sacket's Harbor, at Ogdensburg, at Presque Isle and at Detroit. They did not use Oswego, which was considered unsuitable because of silting, a constant problem that prevented reliable access to and from the shipyards. A yard was established at Black Rock in the Niagara River but, because of problems of defending it, Presque Isle became the principal site for ship construction on Lake Erie.[1] The Canadians had yards at Kingston, York (considered indefensible), Newark and Fort Malden All of these, with the exception of Kingston, were little more than wilderness settlements at the outbreak. Kingston had developed a population of slightly under 1,000 persons.

On Lake Ontario, the Americans had the brig *Oneida*, of 16 guns, plus a number of converted merchantmen. There were at least eight merchantmen at Ogdensburg. Two of these, the *Sophia* and the *Island Packet*, were captured by the British on June 29 and burned. The remaining six, the *Conquest*, the *Growler*, the *Pert*, the *Scourge* and the *Hamilton* were added to the American navy fleet and saw active service.

In the Canadas, British Provincial Marine had, at Kingston, the *Royal George*, a 330-ton, 22-gun ship-rigged vessel (later renamed the *Niagara*), the *Prince Regent* (140 tons, 14 guns) recently finished at York and later named the *General Beresford* and later still, the *Netley*. These were the only two considered fit for service. In addition, there were the *Earl Of Moira* (called the *Elmira* by one writer), the *Duke Of Gloucester* and the *Duke Of Kent*. The latter served as a floating barracks and saw no service whatsoever.

On Lake Erie the Americans had the *Adams*, a brig, being refitted and re-armed at Detroit. She was intended to carry six guns but before they could arrive she was captured by the British on August 16 and renamed the *Detroit*. Lieutenant Jesse D. Elliott, USN, purchased a number of commercial vessels, including the *Amelia* (renamed the *Tigress*), the *Catherine* (renamed the *Somers*) and the *Contractor* (renamed the *Trippe*), and took them into the US Navy

The Provincial Marine, at Fort Malden, had the *Queen Charlotte*, a 16-gun frigate, the *General Hunter*, an old brig of six guns, and a new brig, the *Lady Prevost* with 13 guns, under construction. As well, the North West Company had the *Caledonia* and the *Nancy*, both unarmed transports.

Undoubtedly, the merchant vessels on both sides served as transports or supply-ships, at times, with extra guns. It should be noted that it was customary for merchant vessels, even in times of peace, to carry swivel guns, unsuitable for battle but primarily to be used to discourage possible boarders. Both sides had extremely few professional soldiers or sailors on the lakes. Local militia, largely farmers and tradesmen, were completely untrained and more anxious to get back to their farms to bring in the crops, than to train as soldiers or seamen. Each side had Native allies but they could not be controlled; they were very independent and might fight or they might defect. They were just as apt to ravage the countryside, out of control of the military leaders. Generally, they were more greatly feared by the citizens of both sides than were the regulars – the notable exception was Tecumseh and his men.

There was little enthusiasm for the war in either the militia or the citizenry. Henry Adams wrote later in his account of the war,

"The country refused to take the war seriously."[2] Desertion and defection occurred on both sides. Sir Isaac Brock reported, "...the population, believe me, is essentially bad."[3]

On July 1, the American General William Hull, believing the Canadians near Malden would not yet know that war had been declared, sent an armed schooner, the *Cayahoga*, loaded with stores, personal baggage and official documents on ahead from the mouth of the Maumee River to Detroit. This time the overland mail was intercepted as the *Cayahoga* with General Hull's war plans for the campaign, official mail and much supplies and ordnance was captured by the British at Amherstberg. This vessel was renamed the *Chippewa* and armed with two guns. One writer states that the message that war had been declared, which reached the British first, was one dispatched by Astor to the managers of his fur trading posts at Detroit and Missilimackinac in order to protect his interests in Upper Canada. The message was the first indication to the Canadians at Malden that war had been declared. It made it possible for them to capture Fort Mackinac and Detroit, as well as to take the *Cayahoga*. Oddly, the message was franked[4] by Congress and was obviously sent with the connivance of the American authorities.

Hull invaded Canada at Sandwich (today's Windsor), on July 12 and was amazed to find that the Canadians were not welcoming him with open arms. A few of the Canadian militia defected, perhaps more to save their property than for reasons of allegiance. Two companies of his Michigan Militia deserted. On August 11, Hull withdrew, without attempting to attack Fort Malden. On August 12, the Provincial Marine, using crew and boats from the *Queen Charlotte* and the *General Hunter*, captured an American supply convoy of boats coming from Presque Isle as it headed for Detroit.

Because they had received the news first, the British forces from St. Joseph, on the southern tip of what is now St. Joseph Island, Ontario, using the North West Company's schooner *Caledonia*, captured Fort Mackinac on July 17 without a fight. A small transport loaded with furs from Chicago was also taken. She was the *Friends Good Will*, later named the *Little Belt*. Three others, the *Mary*, the

Erie and the *Salina* were allowed to carry American prisoners back to Cleveland. However, on the way, they landed at Detroit and were captured again by the British when Detroit fell in Brock's fateful attack on August 15. Many of the Michigan Militia deserted and General Hull, fearful of an attack by the Natives, surrendered the town. No British casualties were suffered.

A large quantity of munitions was captured at Detroit on August 15, including cannon, muskets, powder and ball. Some of it was transferred by ship to Fort Erie but was lost to the Americans in a brilliant, cutting-out exercise.[5] However, among the booty were 2,500 American muskets, which the British had kept at Detroit and issued to the local militia. Some of these were still in use up to the end of the war.

On October 9, a party of American soldiers and sailors, under Lieutenant Jesse Elliott USN, cut out two ships near Fort Erie. The *Caledonia* was towed away but the *Detroit* (the former *Adams*) ran aground and had to be burned. This was a daring nighttime exercise that resulted in two vessels being lost by the British and one gained by the Americans. Twenty Americans who had been prisoners were freed, and much of the valuable ordnance captured by the British at Detroit was lost to them. Elliott had only recently arrived at Black Rock, but was the ranking American officer on Lake Erie until Oliver Hazard Perry USN arrived.

On October 13 the American forces invaded Canada at Queenston resulting in the famous Battle of Queenston Heights and the death of the British General Isaac Brock. The Americans were roundly defeated and withdrew with heavy losses. On November 28, they invaded again near Fort Erie and withdrew. The same thing happened on November 30. The commander of these assaults blamed his troops, many of which, he reported, refused to embark or were too fatigued to fight. Thus, at the end of 1812, the Americans had lost two strategic points, Detroit and Mackinac. They had lost their largest vessel on Lake Erie, the *Adams*, and had been repulsed on their invasion attempts at Sandwich, Queenston and Fort Erie.

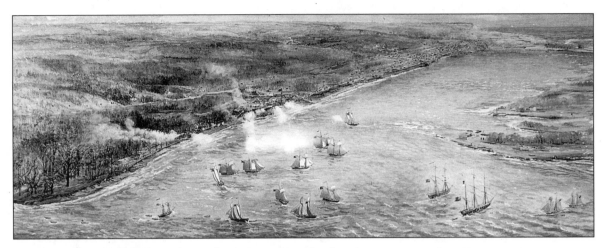

The American fleet attacks York, April 27, 1813, *Owen Staples, artist.* Courtesy of TRL, T10271.

Let us now take a quick look at events on Lake Ontario. On the south shore of the St. Lawrence, the American settlers were definitely opposed to the war. At Ogdensburg, they welcomed their Canadian friends who would cross the river under a flag of truce to shop and to visit. However, sorties of harassment took place. With this part of the country essentially a wilderness, settlers on both sides of the St. Lawrence knew one another, traded back and forth and did not want to fight each other. Friendships and trade continued in spite of the war. Then, at intervals, along would come the army or navy and impose restrictions, but when they went away trade resumed. There are records of both sides in the conflict supplying flour if it was in short supply on the other side and even records of supplying timber for shipbuilding to the other side. Comical in conduct and useless in accomplishment, the official sorties would, at the least, put an end to these friendly visits for the time being.

On November 8, the Americans chased the *Royal George* into the Kingston Harbour but accomplished little other than a demonstration of strength. On the same cruise, they burned a British merchantman loading at the wharf at Ernestown (today's Bath, just west of Kingston, Ontario). The Americans now controlled Lake Ontario and further extended their superiority with the launching of the *Madison*, a 24-gun corvette, at Sacket's Harbor on November 26. The

Provincial Marine had the greater number of ships but was extremely short of trained men. The *Royal George* had only 17 men on board capable of doing their duty and the *Moira* had only ten able seamen.

Britain had been unable to release many seamen or naval officers from the fighting off the coasts of Europe and from blockading the ports of America. However, vessels blockaded in port do not need men and the Americans were thus able to release and dispatch many hundreds of sailors and officers from the Atlantic coastal ports to the lakes as early as the autumn of 1812.

CHAPTER 8

A Shipbuilder's War

The Great Lakes was a self-contained theatre of operations. The ships of the British navy could not help in the war effort. Both sides were dependent on the skills and energies of their men and on the supplies they could accumulate on the scene. Whoever controlled the lakes dominated the supply routes, and vice versa. Without supplies and men, the war was lost. It was only a matter of time!

In the northwest where almost all the fighting took place, it was primarily a naval war, hence a shipbuilder's war. What could Isaac Chauncey, Oliver H. Perry, Thomas Macdonough, Sir James Yeo or Robert Heriot Barclay have accomplished without the ships furnished by the shipyards? Yet, the historians generally give the builders, at most, a few lines in their books, if they mention them at all. Their lives are not well documented. They deserve more attention, but it is difficult to find much about them. They are just as much the heroes of such a war as the commodores, lieutenants, seamen, gunners and other sailors. Shipbuilding, of course, includes the designers, supply officers and administrators, carpenters, caulkers, blacksmiths, rope-makers, riggers, sail makers and labourers, all of whom together as a team of diligent artificers, completed the hasty construction of a ship in the wilderness.

Far more effort went into shipbuilding than all the energy required for the actual fighting on the lakes. It seems, in retrospect, that a great deal of effort went into avoiding battle. After all, the loss of one ship could upset the whole balance of power. The act of conserving one's vessels at all costs was a key strategy. Further, a vessel could be lost in but one hour of intense fighting, yet it had taken all winter to build and would take fully another winter to replace. In the meantime, the war might be lost. As Noah Brown, master shipwright at Presque Isle, said, "We want no extras, plain work, plain work is all we want. They are only required for one battle; if we win that is all that will be wanted of them. If the enemy are victorious, the work is good enough to be captured."

When war was declared, there were only two shipyards of any importance on the lakes, at Kingston and at Fort Malden. They were in a bad state: inefficient, mismanaged and short of supplies and skilled men. But, at least they were established shipyards. On the south shore of Lake Ontario, Oswego had already been declared unsuitable because of silting at its entrance. To serve the Americans on the Upper Lakes, there was only Detroit, and it was of little importance.

The Provincial Marine had not been a proper fighting navy, but primarily a transport service administered by the quartermaster general's department. The ships were manned by "Provincials," a derogatory term applied to these sailors that inferred great inferiority to the men of the Royal Navy. The ships also included some men from the Atlantic Merchant Marine, and a few from among the officers of the Royal Navy. Andrew Grant, commodore on the Upper Lakes, was 78 years old when the war broke out; Captain John Steel, the commander on Lake Ontario was 72. However, the Canadas had more vessels available than the United States on both Lake Ontario and Lake Erie at the outbreak.

To understand the situation in the yard at Kingston, it is necessary to go back a few years. Lieutenant John Schank RN, who had served in the Royal Navy in New England, became commissioner of the lakes after the American Revolution, and served at Kingston from 1778 to 1783. He imported most of his carpenters from British men-of-war and brought his artificers from British dockyards. By 1783 he had over 300 seamen from the British navy serving on the lakes. His entire organization was modelled after Admiralty yards, but none of the officers serving under him was a professional from the Royal Navy. He returned to England in 1785 and many of the British naval and dockyard personnel left also. Possibly some of the Canadian shipwrights, carpenters and other artificers had learned their trades in his shipyard at Carleton Island. Schank was a very forward-thinking and inventive man, in both policies and technology.

While at Lake Champlain in 1776, Schank experimented with the forerunner of the centreboard, the "drop-keel." Twenty years later, it was adopted by the Admiralty for use in shoal-draft vessels around the British coast. It was incorporated into the design of some American schooners as early as 1806, but there is no record of it being used on the lakes during this war. He also experimented with a form of swivel gun that was first introduced in England, in 1798, on the *Wolverine*. She could fight her eight main deck guns on either side, employing athwartship tracks. These were combined with a large circular track on the deck about amidships, as referenced from underwater photographs of wrecks using these devices. It has not been possible to determine how many British ships on the lakes used this invention. Henry Eckford and Noah Brown, at Sacket's Harbor, did arm some vessels this way, notably the *Sylph*. The *Hamilton* is also reported to have been so armed, but perhaps this was after she was acquired by the Americans. Conventional swivel guns were common in both navies. Usually they were small and were mounted on the ships' rails.

At Kingston, in the early 1800s, Silas Pearson had just finished construction of the schooner *Duke Of Kent* when he was dismissed for misappropriation of stores. He was replaced as master shipbuilder by John Dennis, an apparently self-trained boat builder. We know more about him than we do of most of the professional shipbuilders. His family members were successful merchants in Philadelphia, but lost everything in the American Revolutionary War. They owned a piece of property on the banks of the Humber, a few miles northwest of York. Remember that the Humber River was the principal route for

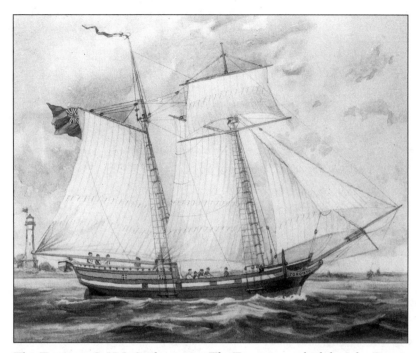

The Toronto, C.H.J. Snider, artist. *The* Toronto *was built by John Dennis in 1799 for government use. She carried passengers and government dispatches all along the Canadian shores of Lake Ontario. She was wrecked on Toronto Island.* Courtesy of TRL, T15210.

transporting men and equipment to Lake Simcoe and Georgian Bay, carrying furs on the return trip. The Dennis property eventually became the Toronto suburb of Mount Dennis, though it would be difficult to find on a Toronto map today. Dennis had a shipyard at the mouth of the Humber and among the vessels built there in 1798 was the *Toronto*, a schooner, built for the use of government officials. She was wrecked on Toronto Island in 1801.

Dennis was master shipwright for many of the ships built on Lake Ontario in the early 1800s: the *Earl Of Moira*, (14 guns) 1805 (renamed the *Charwell* in 1813); the *Duke Of Gloucester*, May, 1806; the *Royal George*, (20 guns), July, 1809; the *Prince Regent*, (8 guns), July 1812, (renamed *General Beresford*); and for the *Sir Isaac Brock*, burned by the British, unfinished in the stocks at her shipyard in York, 1813, during the American attack. She was thus prevented from falling into

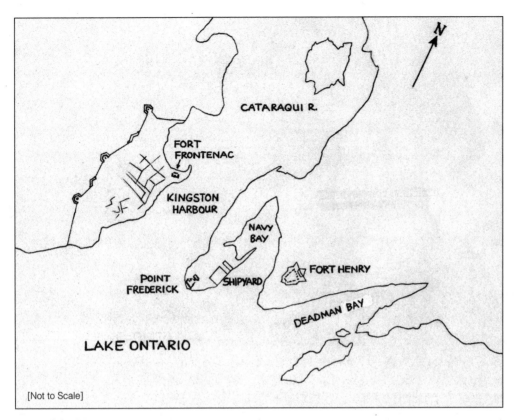

Map of the Kingston area, 1812. Sketch by Heidi Hoffman.

American hands. It is interesting to note that during this period, 1812, Captain Andrew Gray,[1] the quartermaster general beginning in 1811, reported on the shortage of the workforce to Sir George Prevost, Governor General of Canada, "the want of seamen is so great that the *Royal George* has only 17 men and the *Moira* only 10 able seamen."

The fleet at Kingston at the outset of the war included *Earl Of Moira*, built at Kingston, 1805 (169 ton, 14 guns); *Sir Sidney Smith*, built at Kingston, 1806 (37 ton, 14 guns); *Duke Of Gloucester* built at Kingston, 1807 (6 guns); *Royal George* built at Kingston, 1809 (330 ton, 22 guns); *Prince Regent* built at York, 1812 (141 ton, 16 guns). Before the 1813 sailing season commenced, on April 28, the *Sir George Prevost* was launched and immediately renamed the *Wolfe*. At the time the names of ships were frequently changed, sometimes for unknown reason. Seemingly, it is customary in the Royal Navy never to name a ship after a living monarch or high official – perhaps it was considered bad luck.[2] There were also several merchant schooners used for transports, some of which had been captured from the Americans.

After a period of time in Kingston, John Dennis had moved back to York where he was working on the *Sir Isaac Brock* when the Americans attacked. As noted earlier, the *Brock* was burned in her stocks to prevent her from falling into American hands.

In the Canadian shipyards, as 1812 drew to a close, it was a case of make do with whatever was available, sometimes with drastic results. Essentially all supplies had to be supplied from England via Quebec and Montreal, and then overland to Kingston. Guns and stores were commandeered from ships and forts at Halifax, Quebec and Montreal and forwarded on to Kingston There was an iron foundry at Quebec but there is no record of it doing any work for the vessels under construction on the lakes.

Initially, there was no shortage of timber around any of the shipyards. Forests of oak, pine, chestnut, cedar, walnut, ash and other species were near at hand. Fortunately, the majority of the settlers were skilled axe men. However, shortages of oak timber showed up before the war ended. Along the Detroit River near the yard at Fort Malden, there was a ropewalk (a facility where rope is made) where rope and cable could be produced from locally grown hemp. There may have been other walks in the Canadas, but most of the rope and cable was imported from England at the time.

On December 28, 1812, a group of some 130 shipwrights, carpenters and other artisans arrived at Kingston, gathered from the yards in Montreal and Quebec. They were distributed among the shipyards and the building pace picked up, though not without difficulties. At Kingston, a new master builder, James Morrison, was discharged as incompetent. He was replaced by Daniel Allen who, in turn, was soon discharged for being the "primary cause of the little discontents which have been manifested by the artificers"[3] in a dockyard strike. The yards did have their personnel problems.

On April 26, 1813, Isaac Chauncey appeared off York with his fleet, consisting of the *Oneida*, the *Madison* and gunboats. Major

General Dearborn was on board, along with Brigadier General Zebulon Pike and some 1,700 troops. The American commanders determined that Kingston was too well guarded for it to be attacked with reasonable chance of success, but York was virtually undefended. Although York had little military significance, it was on the supply line to the Niagara Peninsula and Amherstburg. Also, the *Prince Regent* was reported to be there, and should be easily captured with the force he had at his disposal. York was the capital of Upper Canada. Its destruction would be a major morale booster for the Americans, if it could be accomplished, and most dispiriting for the British.

Although the small fort was soon demolished by the American invaders, the powder magazine at Fort York was set to be blown up by the British defenders as they escaped. In the massive explosion that followed, there was great loss of life to the American invaders, including that of Brigadier General Pike. They lost 320 men, killed or wounded.

Although the *Prince Regent* had already left York and was sailing to Kingston on the 24th of April, the Americans were able to acquire large quantities of naval and military stores, all captured at York. These were either taken or destroyed, including the cannons and other materials that Robert Barclay needed so badly at Fort Malden.

On May 1, the parliament buildings at York were set on fire under mysterious circumstances. Some have blamed the American soldiers, but it appears that is incorrect. The blame is now assigned to recent immigrants from the United States who had maintained loyalty to their former home.[4] Could it be that these arsonists were planted in Upper Canada by American strategists to take advantage of such an opportunity?

The *Duke of Gloucester*, undergoing repairs in York, was captured by the Americans. She was in a poor state and of little value, so was torched. A Canadian merchant schooner, the *Governor Hunter*, was also burned but Major-General Henry Dearborn paid the owner $300, on the spot, using money confiscated from the public treasury. Dearborn reported taking "no vessel fit for use." Many private homes in York were looted, along with merchants' stores.

From a military point of view the actions made no sense. It seems to have been a case of getting even, but such acts of vandalism

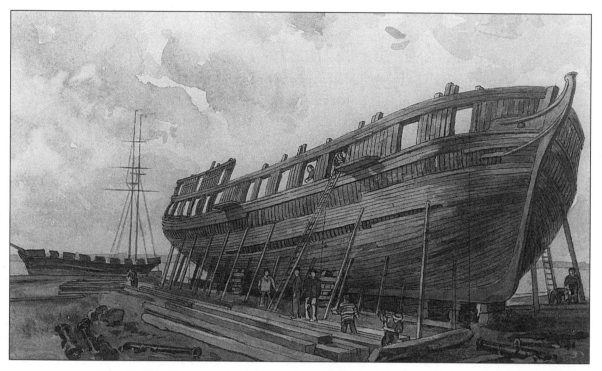

The Sir Isaac Brock *under construction at York, April 1813. C.H.J. Snider, artist.* Courtesy of TRL T15211.

and retaliation were perpetrated by both sides. The Americans burned the village of Newark on December 13, putting the inhabitants out into the cold. The British, in retaliation, burned Buffalo and five of Perry's ships on December 27. The Americans wiped out the unarmed village of Port Dover on Lake Erie in April 1814. If the Americans could destroy the capital of Upper Canada, the British could retaliate by burning Washington. Such was the excuse given for the attack on Washington the following August.

Commander Chauncey did not know it, but by his actions at York, he had determined the course of the war on Lake Erie. He had captured all the cannon intended for arming the new ship being built for Barclay at Fort Malden. This certainly was a principal cause of the disastrous defeat in the Battle of Lake Erie on September 10, 1813. York had been considered indefensible from the outset. But why, then, were large ships being built at the yards there? Apparently, it was a political decision, the intention being to spread the largesse around and to provide employment to the community. The workers repaid with labor unrest and strikes. Had the work proceeded as quickly as it could have, the *Brock* might have been finished, instead of being lost.

On March 19, 1813, Captain Sir James Lucas Yeo, RN, was appointed commodore and commander-in-chief of British navy operations on the Great Lakes. He was 30 years old and a veteran of many actions. He had gone to sea at the age of ten and was elevated to the rank of post-captain at 25. Upon his arrival at Kingston on May 15, he soon found out that the squadron was in a very weak state and the enemy in a much superior position. The *Sir Isaac Brock*, which the British needed badly, had been burned at York in the previous month, April 27. Yeo brought with him three commanders, eight lieutenants, two pursers, two master mates, eighteen midshipmen and 400 seamen. These men could only serve as a nucleus for the existing ships and the ships to be constructed, but it was certainly a good start.

Among the officers arriving at this time was Lieutenant Robert Barclay, 28, who had fought under Lord Nelson at the Battle of Trafalgar. He, like Nelson, had lost an arm in another engagement. Barclay was to take command of the fleet at Fort Malden and had arrived there June 7. At this point, control over the Provincial Marine was transferred to Commodore Yeo. It became part of the Royal Navy on June 24, 1813. Along with Yeo was Captain Richard O'Conor, who was to take charge of the shore establishments, crew and shipbuilding operations. A competent dockyard superintendent, he had received his earlier experience at Woolwich, Deptford and Portsmouth yards in England. With him arrived more shipwrights and carpenters. With these reinforcements, shipbuilding was able to progress much faster in the yards both at Kingston and Malden. No more ships for the war were built at York.

On the American side, the decision was taken, early on, to abandon Oswego as a shipbuilding site and to build at Sacket's Harbor in the southeast corner of Lake Ontario. It was the only really good harbour on the south shore, being deep and relatively easy to defend. Lieutenant Melancthon Woolsey was sent to Sacket's in 1809 to take charge and arrange for the building of the *Oneida*. Both Henry Eckford, master shipwright, USN, and Christian Bergh, one of his shipwrights, came up from New York with additional carpenters and artisans to take charge of the actual construction. When finished, the *Oneida* was armed with 16 guns. The reported cost of building the vessel was $20,505.00 and 110 gallons of liquor.

In the spring of 1812, Woolsey bought a number of merchant ships, all of which he armed, including the *Diana*, and captured the *Lord Nelson*. She was carrying a load of flour and other freight from Prescott to Niagara when seized, two weeks before war was declared. The *Lord Nelson* was taken to Sacket's and refitted as a warship and renamed the *Scourge*. They, plus the *Oneida*, constituted the American navy on Lake Ontario when war was declared. Woolsey was ordered to start construction of a corvette of the same general dimensions as the *Royal George*, and it was well underway when Chauncey arrived at Sacket's Harbor in September. On November 26, the 24-gun corvette, *Madison*, was launched. She had been built in the amazingly short period of 45 days by Henry Eckford. Of her, Chauncey wrote, "...a beautiful corvette-built ship" of 540 tons, "nine weeks before, the timber of which she was constructed was growing in the woods." The fleet at Sacket's then consisted of the *Oneida*, the *Madison*, and six armed merchant vessels. The *Hamilton* (ex *Diana*) and the *Scourge* (ex *Lord Nelson*) were among them.

In September 1812, Captain Isaac Chauncey was ordered, by the Secretary of the Navy Paul Hamilton, to take command of the American naval forces on the lakes. He had been the officer in charge of the Brooklyn Navy Yards and had served in America's wars with France and Tripoli.[5] He made his base at Sacket's Harbor, but before leaving Washington himself, he had dispatched a force of shipwrights, artisans, seamen and marines, along with a hundred cannon and much ordnance, cordage, sails and building materials, chain, spikes, bolts and other iron work to the shipyard there.

In January of the next year, William Jones became Secretary of the Navy, replacing Hamilton. He had great confidence in Chauncey but emphasized their strategy in a letter to the commodore, dated January

27, "It is impossible to attach too much importance to our naval operations on the Lakes – the success … will depend absolutely on our superiority on all the Lakes."[6] He virtually gave Chauncey carte blanche and a blank cheque – "Whatever force the Enemy may create, we must surpass."

Chauncey hired Henry Eckford as his chief designer and constructor. A Scot of 37 years who had learned the trade at the shipyards in Quebec, Eckford served some time in the Provincial Marine, then moved to New York City. There he earned a reputation of being a top designer. Eckford-built vessels were recognized as ones that reliably and dependably surpassed rivals in stability, speed and capacity. His efforts were concentrated at the Sacket's Harbor yard but, along with Chauncey, he visited Presque Isle on December 31. During that one-day visit, he changed the designs of two brigs under construction, giving them a particularly shallow draft so that they could cross the sandbar at the mouth of the harbour. He also suggested changes in two of the gunboats that were under construction at the time of the visit, and had a hand in designing the modifications of the merchant ships being converted to gunboats at Black Rock. After the war, in the 1820s, he spent his final years in Turkey building ships-of-the-line for the Turkish Navy. He died there in 1832.

There had been an attempt to establish a shipyard at Black Rock, near the entrance of the Niagara River but it was abandoned, being too near the guns of Fort Erie. Several merchant ships were rebuilt here but they could not join Perry at Presque Isle until after Fort Erie had been captured. Daniel Dobbins had been appointed to take charge of shipbuilding on Lake Erie in September 1811. A local settler and trader, and a ship owner Dobbins lived at Erie, and knew the lake well but was not a master shipwright. (He was one of those captured by the British when they took Mackinac on July 17, 1812 but was released along with his ship, the *Salina*, to take prisoners back to Cleveland.) Immediately after his appointment, he started procuring materials and hired a shipwright named Ebenezer Crosby to assist in the work both at Black Rock and at Presque Isle. Crosby played a major part in the management of the work, designing, supervising and actually working on the physical construction of the ships. However, when Noah Brown, who had been hired by Chaucey to take charge of the site, arrived in March 1813, Crosby disappears from the records.

One morning in February 1813, Dobbins spied a ship in the ice some ten miles off the shipyard at Erie. He had the men rig up two horse-drawn sleighs. Taking a party with him, they drove out on the ice to examine the vessel. There lay the lost *Salina*! It had been captured again by the British off Fort Malden and the load of prisoners had been sent on, presumably on foot, Dobbin later learned that it had stuck in the ice off Malden and the crew had deserted the ship and walked to shore across the ice. The *Salina* had slowly drifted down to Lake Erie and ultimately fetched up in the heavy pack ice off the Presque Isle shipyard. Dobbins and his men were able to salvage a load of frozen food, rigging, cables, ropes, and about 6,000 pounds of iron fittings, cannon balls and anchors. Then, to prevent her falling into the hands of the British again, the *Salina* was burned.

Noah Brown was the one man most responsible for the physical work done on the American ships at Presque Isle. In 1804, with his brother Adam, he built his first vessel, a schooner named *Work* for the North West Company, at Newark on the Niagara River. Noah then moved to New York City where he operated a shipyard with his brother, either adjacent to that of Henry Eckford or shared with Eckford. Chauncey hired Brown in New York in February 1813 and sent him up to Erie where he arrived on February 24. Brother Adam remained in New York to operate the yard there and to help find men and supplies for Noah. On arrival at Presque Isle, Noah immediately assumed the position of superintendent of construction. Initially there were some shortages of labour at the yard, but by May two hundred men were working there and the construction of vessels was proceeding at a fast pace.

It wasn't long before labour difficulties presented another set of problems. Just as an angry crew could suddenly "strike" (drop) the sails to make a point with a demanding captain, the shipyard at Presque Isle also experienced labour strikes as a result of shortages of food for the men and more problems in getting all the materials needed for the vessels under construction. At times iron was in very short supply, but towards the end of the ship building era, following the Battle of Lake Erie in 1813, they were cutting up iron to fill leather bags of scrap, which could be fired at the rigging of the British vessels when they came into close range. People at Presque Isle suffered much from an illness they called "bilious remitting fever," which kept many workers, soldiers and seamen on the sick list. Even Captain Perry, based there as officer in charge, was not immune to the affliction.

Brown left Presque Isle late in July 1813 before the ships were rigged, leaving his foreman, Sidney Wright, and sixteen carpenters to finish up. In the period from February 10 to September 10, he had built the 260-ton ships, the *Lawrence* and the *Niagara*; a 75-ton schooner, *Ariel*; gunboat schooners, *Ohio*, *Porcupine* and *Scorpion*; and had rebuilt the *Tigress*. In addition, he built four camels, 50 feet long, 10 feet wide and 8 feet deep.[7] These were used to lift the larger, deep draft vessels over the bar in the harbour entrance. In a short time, in a wilderness setting, he had accomplished miracles.

After completion of the work at Erie, Noah and Adam took charge of the construction of ships for Thomas Macdonaugh, the commander of the US fleet on Lake Champlain. Next they went to Sacket's Harbor to work on the two 130-gun first-raters[8] with Henry Eckford, taking 1,200 workers with them. This was in February 1815, but they only worked there for six weeks when the declaration of peace put an end to their labours in the wilderness. Noah returned to New York where he continued to build ships and naval fortifications He lived and worked up to the age of seventy, but died in poverty. Henry Eckford, Noah and Adam Brown had proven to be outstanding builders, heroes of the Battle of Lake Erie just as much as was Captain Oliver Hazard Perry.

Perry was only 27 when appointed to take charge of the naval forces on Lake Erie on February 5, 1813. Born in Rhode Island, he had joined the navy at the age of 13 as midshipman under his father, Captain Christopher Raymond Perry, and served in Europe and North America. At the age of 20 he was promoted to lieutenant with a small schooner under his command. By 1812, he was master commandant and given command of twelve gunboats operating off the Connecticut shores. Apparently this action was not exciting enough for him and he requested service on the Great Lakes. Immediately following his new appointment, he dispatched three groups of fifty seamen to the lakes before heading there himself. He spent a few weeks at Sacket's before proceeding to Erie, arriving there on March 27.

From then until August he was continually on the move, obtaining supplies and men anywhere they could be found. Undoubtedly, Perry's energetic efforts in solving almost insurmountable problems of supply and labour were as great a contribution to the project as his leadership in the battle. Through his efforts, the ships were built, armed and manned quickly. Without them, the situation on Lake Erie could have been quite different. Both Chauncey, at Sacket's Harbor, and Perry, at Erie, had the advantage of access to skilled tradesmen. Their supply routes, which were generally safe from interruption, provided easier access to a native industry in Pittsburg and to goods from other communities. They had access to men and materials that could be spared from ships blockaded in Atlantic ports. Even though the roads were choked all winter, sleighs continued hauling supplies to Sacket's Harbor, Black Rock and Erie.

In a letter to President Madison on October 26, 1814, Secretary of the Navy Jones wrote that the British "may transport without interruption from the Ocean to Lake Ontario, at less time, and at one fourth of the expense, that we can transport from Washington to New York." This was obviously totally wrong. The cost of shipping from England to Kingston, let alone the time it took, was extreme. It cost £2,000 to transport six 32-pounders from Quebec to Kingston and £4,000 to transport forty 24-pounders from Montreal to Kingston. Canadian yards and forces had far greater supply problems for both material and personnel. Two hundred ox-teams and drivers were hired from Vermont and New Hampshire to haul cannon and other supplies on this route.

At Amherstburg Major General Henry Proctor was in command and Captain George B. Hall was superintendent of the dockyard.

William Bell, a Scotsman from Leith who learned his trade in the yards at Quebec, had been building vessels there since 1799 and was master shipwright when Robert Barclay arrived.

Bell had built the snow, *Camden*, in 1804, but it was declared unfit to go to sea in 1812. He built the *Queen Charlotte* in 1809 and the *Lady Prevost* in 1812. Two gunboats, the *Myers* and the *Eliza* were launched in March 1813, and the corvette, *Detroit*, (a new *Detroit*) was under construction. The *General Hunter*, built in 1806, was declared "fast falling into decay." The schooner, *Nancy*, was commandeered from the North West Company for use as a transport. Early in July, the *Chippewa* (built in 1810 on the Maumee River, which flows into Lake Erie at the extreme western tip), was captured as well as the *Friends Good Will* (later renamed *Little Belt* as noted earlier) and the *Cayahoga Packet*. These vessels were part of the British fleet when Barclay arrived.

There were always shortages at Amherstburg. Bell was forced to cannibalize the old *Camden* in order to get her iron for the other vessels under construction. Although work on the new vessel had the highest priority, Barclay reported that, when repairs were needed for one of the others, work temporarily stopped on the *Detroit*. Barclay made repeated requests for more shipwrights, artisans, seamen, munitions and other supplies but was met with very little but promises. Commodore Yeo needed every able-bodied man he could get for his own building program at Kingston and could spare very few for Barclay. When pressured by Barclay for guns, he responded, "…the ordnance and Naval stores you require must be taken from the enemy whose resources on Lake Erie must become yours." The guns intended for the *Detroit* had been captured by the Americans when they attacked York in April. Despite all obstacles, the *Detroit* was launched on July 12, though neither munitions nor men had arrived. After the battle, William Bell moved to the Kingston shipyard and is credited with the speedy construction of the *St. Lawrence*. In mid-April 1813, the *Wolfe* was launched at Kingston and shortly after, the *Lord Melville*, but there were not enough sailors to operate these ships.

On June 12, 1813, Eckford launched the *General Pike* (26 guns) at Sacket's and started the *Sylph*. At Presque Isle, Perry's fleet was about ready for action by the first of August.

Success in constructing and arming adequate lake navies stood in vivid contrast to the failure that was experienced in staffing and training the crews. No one, however, can ever claim any credit for adequately crewing and arming the *Detroit* even though she was built in good time. Trained seamen were not sent to Amherstburg for her crew and, as noted, her cannon were lost when Chauncey attacked York. In fact, Barclay was forced to scavenge land cannon from the fort and to acquire guns from other vessels. Records show that there were Native members of the crew and that one of his smaller ships was crewed by untrained teenagers. Loss of the cannon was probably the principal reason for defeat in the Battle of Lake Erie in 1813. Barclay was severely criticized for attempting battle without his proper cannon, but he had no alternative and was completely exonerated at the court martial back in London, England.

CHAPTER 9

The Lake Ontario Theatre in 1813–14

On Lake Ontario, both sides seemed to want to avoid a decisive battle. Should Commodore Yeo have lost a major part of his fleet, the Americans would have had a free hand in taking over Upper Canada. They would have gained the ability to move down to attack Montreal. If Commodore Chauncey had lost part of his fleet, it could only have delayed the outcome, not changed it, providing the war continued, which of course it did not. Peace was declared on December 24, 1814.

When the 1813 navigation season ended, shipbuilding proceeded as fast as possible on both sides of Lake Ontario in spite of many difficulties. Yeo wrote to the Governor General Prevost on December 2, 1813, "I have no doubt Your Excellency will agree with me that great military advantage may be obtained by our squadron being on the lake three weeks or a month before that of the enemy, which from the forward state of the new ships, I think likely. They are, however, of a size and force that will require a large complement of men, particularly the large one, which if properly appointed, will exceed any frigate in the British navy. I deem it my duty to assure Your Excellency that great credit is due to Captain [Richard] Conor for his very zealous exertions in the dockyard. Both ships are in a very forward state and everything goes on with a spirit that is highly satisfactory."' Both ships, the *Princess Charlotte* and the *Prince Regent* were launched on April 14, 1814, and would need 550 seamen.

Thomas Strickland was master shipwright about this time. He had served at shipyards at Plymouth and Portsmouth and other yards in England. He knew his profession intimately and his name appears on the draughts of several ships, notably the *St. Lawrence*. (His career was cut short by a riding accident in September 1815, which resulted in his death.)

The British were learning to arm their new vessels with more long guns and fewer carronades, (the cannons that fired large projectiles, but which were effective only for short range). The guns had to be hauled up from Quebec on sleighs during the winter, a major task and a very expensive one.

Both shipyards had labour problems. The several superintendents and master builders who had to be replaced at Kingston and the strike there have already been mentioned. In another incident, 14 shipwrights absconded, but were arrested and forced to return to work. At Sacket's Harbor, on May 2, 1813, there was a riot in the yard. Shipwrights and carpenters, armed with axes and adzes attacked a group of soldiers "brandishing their weapons in the wildest frenzy of rage." Fortunately, Henry Eckford, Isaac Chauncey and Noah Brown intervened and persuaded the antagonists to desist and to return to work.

Chauncey attacked Presqu'île (Upper Canada) at the end of June and destroyed a schooner under construction. Presqu'île saw several similar events, and appears to have been undefended. On one occasion an expedition of Americans landed and intercepted the mails thereby obtaining military dispatches and strategic plans of great importance. On another occasion, June 16, 1813, Lieutenant Wolcott Chauncey, Commander Chauncey's brother, cruising in the *Lady of the Lake*, captured the British *Lady Murray* and took the prize into Sacket's. During another attack on Presqu'île in July 1814, the British captured an American boat after a sharp exchange in which half the

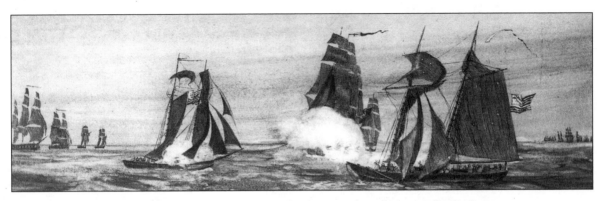

The capture of the American schooners, USS Julia *and* USS Growler *off Niagara by Sir James Lucas Yeo's squadron on August 10, 1813. The* Julia *is in the forefront to the left and the* Growler *to the right. They were renamed the* Confiance *and the* Hamilton. *The ships changed hands again in October 1813 and the* Growler *was recaptured by the British in May 1814. C.H.J. Snider, artist.* Courtesy of TRL., John Ross Robertson Collection, Ref. No. 1149.

crew were killed or wounded. The prize turned out to be Yeo's own gig, the light, narrow, speedy ship's boat, often reserved for the captain's use. It had been lost at Sandy Creek.

The British attempted an in-the-water "frog-man" attack at Sacket's on April 25, 1813. The attack was thwarted, but the Americans discovered several small kegs of powder on the beach the following morning, thus verifying what was intended. Similarly, Chauncey sent a midshipman in a barge, with a "torpedo" to enter Kingston harbour and blow up the *St. Lawrence*, but this attempt also was foiled.

Chauncey had launched his two frigates, the *Superior* and the *Mohawk* on May 1 and June 11,1813, respectively, and he attacked York for the second time on July 31, 1813. Seemingly no real fighting took place other than a "war of words," with Reverend John Strachan[2] actively engaged in the exchange. Some looting occurred, but talking prevailed.

All these incidents and skirmishes were of relatively little value, serving to disrupt and annoy rather than to play a decisive role in the war. Several times smaller ships changed hands. The American ships, *Julia* and *Growler* were taken by the British on August 9, 1813, and renamed *Confiance* and *Hamilton*. But they were recaptured by the

Americans on October 5, almost before the paint had a chance to dry. Actually, storms did as much damage as naval action, witness the loss of the *Hamilton* and *Scourge* in a squall in August 1813.

Another example of the perils of tempestuous weather, although not specifically related to our story of sail, occurred in late 1813. In August of that year, John Armstrong, the American Secretary of War, started plans to assault Kingston. It was October before the plans were executed. Major General James Wilkinson, elderly and in poor health, was placed in charge. On October 17, the expedition set out from Sacket's Harbor in wintery weather. The force consisted of eight thousand soldiers and officers in 300 bateaux with twelve of Chauncey's fleet of gunboats to defend them. Before the fleet had even reached Grenadier Island, only eighteen miles from Sacket's Harbor, a severe storm with driving wind and heavy rain hammered the fleet. Many boats were driven ashore and wrecked. Military supplies and provisions were soaked and destroyed, and a third of their rations were lost. "The morning disclosed a scene of desolation truly distressing," wrote Franklin B. Hough in his book, *History of Jefferson County in the State of New York from the Earliest Time to the Present Time*. "The shores of the island and mainland were strewn with broken and sunken boats."[3] Many of the soldiers became sick and had to be sent back to Sacket's. It was the 28th of October before they could depart from Grenadier Island.

Even though they were close to Kingston, Wilkinson changed his mind and decided to proceed down the St. Lawrence and to attack Montreal. They finally got themselves organized and under way, but then learned that they were under pursuit by a small fleet of British gunboats from Kingston. The British caught up with them by November 10, near Chrysler's farm in Upper Canada. Wilkinson, quite ill by this time, decided to make a stand here. His campaign was doomed from the start. At Chrysler's farm, on November 11, in pitched battle, the straggling American forces were defeated by eight hundred British regulars and Canadian militia, with help from the gunboats from Kingston.

Wilkinson retreated to Fort Covington (currently Covington, New York, across the St. Lawrence from Cornwall, Ontario) with the remnants of his troops, his career over. Pierre Berton recounts this disaster very well in his book, *Flames Across the Border*. As a matter of general interest, the well-known Warden of the Forest, Dr. William "Tiger" Dunlop,[4] of the Canada Company-Huron Tract fame, was an assistant surgeon in the 89th at this time. He helped to look after the wounded of both sides in this infamous battle.

On land, following the Battle of Lake Erie, the British abandoned Detroit on September 24, 1813. Similarly, they left Fort Malden two days later, then withdrew up the Thames Valley to Moravian Town. The American army, under Major General William Henry Harrison, accompanied by Perry, invaded Canada on the Detroit frontier and followed the retreating troops. The British suffered a major defeat with great loss of life, then withdrew what forces were left to the west end of Lake Ontario in the vicinity of present-day Burlington Heights. Harrison retreated to the Detroit River, then sailed with Perry to Buffalo leaving troops to garrison Detroit, Sandwich and Amherstburg. Most of his troops were transported to Buffalo and then, after crossing to Lake Ontario, Chauncey took them to Sacket's Harbor.

On the Niagara frontier, the American Brigadier General George McClure could not hold on to the land being occupied, that small part of the Niagara Peninsula including Newark (now Niagara-on-the-Lake), as the New York Militia refused to serve beyond its specified commitment and went home. McClure withdrew, burning the village of Newark (December 10, 1813) on the way. At the time, the commanders of the land forces on both sides complained about lack of cooperation from the navy. With no unified command in those days, both the army and navy operated independently.

Chauncey was accused by his superiors of disobeying orders and there were even intimations of cowardice. His ship, the *Superior*, was launched on May 1, 1814, but did not leave Sacket's Harbor until August 1. Actually, he had labour troubles in his yard with about half of his men sick with the bilious remitting fever. He too was ill for a short time, but wars do not usually stop because a high-ranking officer is not well. It was said of him that he treated the fleet as if it were his own personal property, not that of the government.

On August 10, Chauncey wrote to General Jacob Brown, who was in charge of the land forces attacking on the Niagara frontier:

> That you might find the fleet somewhat of a convenience in the transportation of provisions and stores for the use of the army and an agreeable appendage to attend its marches and countermarches, I am ready to believe, but, Sir, the Secretary of the Navy has honoured me with a higher destiny – we are intended to seek and to destroy the enemy's fleet. This is the great purpose of the government in creating this fleet and I shall not be diverted in my efforts to effectuate it by any sinister attempt to render us subordinate to or an appendage of the army.[5]

Chauncey was not about to share his naval forces with any land-based forces.

On August 5, the Secretary of the Navy William Jones, being most unhappy with Chauncey's performance, had ordered Captain Stephen Decatur[6] to take command of Lake Ontario and replace the wayward naval commander. The order was revoked, however, when it was learned that Chauncey had already started to act. He effectively took control of the lake, blockading York and Niagara until the *St. Lawrence* was launched by the British at Kingston on September 21, and was ready to go to sea on October 15. Although the fleets rarely aided the armies by carrying troops and supplies, they did provide substantial assistance by preventing the other side from doing the same.

On the morning of August 5, 1814, the American fleet, the *Sylph*, *Jefferson* and *Oneida*, intercepted the British *Magnet*, bound from York to Niagara with a detachment of troops. She was forced to run aground near the mouth of Ten Mile Creek, some ten miles from the mouth of the Niagara River, to avoid capture. The brig *Sylph* was ordered to work her way in close to shore and destroy the *Magnet* or take her as a prize. Before this could be done, however, the stranded *Magnet* was torched by her own crew and soon blew up.

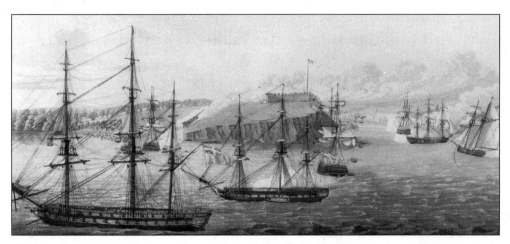

*The British attack on Oswego on May 6, 1814, from a drawing by Lieutenant John Hewett.
In the foreground is* HMS Prince Regent. Courtesy of Library and Archives Canada, C794.

After Napoleon abdicated in April 1814 and was exiled, more British sailors, soldiers and marines became available for transport to Canada. About the same time, the crews of American ships, blockaded in Atlantic ports, were sent up to Chauncey for his use. Officers, ordinary seamen and marines of the US Congress were released for Great Lakes duty under orders from Secretary of the Navy Jones on May 31, 1814.

Both sides made attacks on villages along the enemy's shore but each made certain they would not be involved in any decisive engagement. The British attacked the American Fort Ontario (today in Oswego, New York, at the mouth of the Oswego River) on May 6, 1814, but only after considerable delay due to bad weather. They captured the fort but suffered considerable loss of men, wounded or killed. In the little cemetery near the fort, one can still see several gravestones in memory of British forces who died in the battle.

The delay had permitted the Americans to move most of their military stores up the Oswego River to safety. Many of the buildings in both the fort and in the village were burned. Commodore Yeo withdrew and returned to Kingston on May 7 with minimal booty but did recapture the *Growler*. He declared the enterprise a "compleat victory." However, the Americans were able to retain most of their munitions and stores intended for relocation to Sacket's. Yeo attempted to capture the military stores being transferred by water from Oswego to Sacket's on May 29, but the attack was only partly successful. The British troops followed the Americans up Sandy Creek, eight miles west of Sacket's, but were ambushed. Several gunboats were lost (including Yeo's gig) and many of the British were killed, wounded, or taken prisoner.

Just how fortunate Yeo was in the winter of 1813-14 is demonstrated by recounting that new sails for these ships, in fact every sail the squadron possessed, were nearly lost when a fire broke out in a barrack room above the sail loft. The fire was extinguished but it came closer to destroying the balance of power on Lake Ontario than anything Chauncey ever did. It could have been another case of "for want of a nail… the war was lost."

Captain Robert Hall RN (later Sir Robert Hall) took up the post of commissioner at Kingston in October, 1814, and Captain Conor returned to England with reports from Yeo to the British Admiralty.

In spite of these incidents and circumstances, the shipbuilders' war went on. Yeo succeeded on launching the *St. Lawrence* in Kingston on September 21, 1814. But before she was ready to go to sea on October 15, Chauncey removed his entire fleet from the dangers on Lake Ontario into the relative security of the harbour at Sacket's, knowing full well that he had no ship that could match the *St. Lawrence*. They never ventured forth again during the war.

The British fleet at the end of hostilities included:

	Tons	Guns
St. Lawrence	2305	102
Kingston	1294	58
Burlington, ex *Charlotte*	756	44
Psyche	769	56
Star, ex *Lord Melville*	186	14
Montreal, ex *Wolfe*	426	23
Niagara, ex *Royal George*	330	21
Netley, ex *Beresford*	7	12
Charwell, ex *Earl of Moira*	?	13
Plus gun-ships and transports		

When news of peace arrived on the lakes, the British had two more ships-of-the-line under construction at Kingston. They were to be called the *Canada* and the *Wolfe*, each to be of 2,152 tons. They had been started but were never finished. In addition, frames for three vessels had been made in England and shipped out for assembly and ultimate use on the Great Lakes. The *Psyche*, one of the kits, was actually finished in December 1814. She was sent over from England in pieces, along with all her rigging, guns and other equipment. The freight charges for her timbers just from Quebec to Kingston, exceeded £12,000.[7] The Lords of the Admiralty either did not know, or forgot, that the Great Lakes were freshwater bodies. "A large supply of water casks accompanied them although it was only necessary to drop a bucket alongside, to get up as much as wanted, and that of an excellent quality," wrote John Duncan in his book, *Travels Through the United States and Canada in 1818-19.*[8]

At the same time, the American fleet consisted of:

	Tons	Guns
Superior	1580	58
Mohawk	1350	42
Madison	875	26
General Pike	875	26
Jefferson	500	20
Jones	500	20
Oneida	?	17
Governor Tomkins	?	16
Sylph	?	14
Lady Of The Lake	?	?

Plus various gunboats and transports

Isaac Chauncey had two line-of-battle ships under construction. They were the *Chippewa* and the *New Orleans*, each to be 1,748 tons and 100 guns. They were never launched. I am only speculating here but could one of them be armed with the cannon that had been shipped from England intended for Barclay's *Detroit*? These cannon

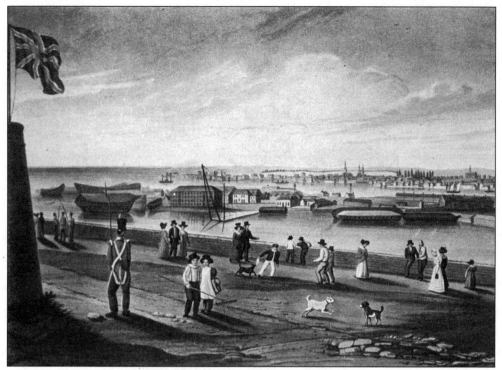

Naval Dockyard at Point Frederick, 1815. *E.E. Vidal, artist. Navy Bay is in the middle ground.* Courtesy of Massey College, Royal Military College, Kingston, Ontario.

had been captured when Chauncey attacked York in April 1813. Reports show a great deal of military stores were taken but nothing further is heard about all those cannon. All in all, there are great differences in how various authors, and even the official Navy returns, describe the ships and their armaments.

By the mid-1850s, the railways were extending into the country where there was commercial timber to be cut and taken to market. The lumber trade reached its peak in the 1880s and the sailing fleets reached their peak in the same period, though it didn't die out completely until almost all the ships had passed their lifespan and steam-powered ships had proven cheaper to operate, and more reliable.

With them went the last of the freshwater crews that had hauled at anchor cables, pulled at the halyards and sheets, steered, loaded and unloaded cargo and raised their voices together.[9]

CHAPTER 10

Comments on the Battle of Lake Erie

ACTUALLY, THERE WAS ONLY ONE BATTLE of real importance on the Great Lakes during the war. The story of the Battle of Lake Erie has been written many, many times, but some of the earlier stories are more propaganda than fact. A good example of the exaggerations can be found in *The Naval War of 1812*, written by President Theodore Roosevelt, in part while he was a student at Princeton. (One of the more recent, and from my perspective, perhaps among the best accounts of the battle because of style and excellent notes, is *HMS Detroit: The Battle for Lake Erie* by Robert and Thomas Malcolmson.)

On the day of battle, September 10, 1813, the fleet under the command of Captain Oliver Hazard Perry USN consisted of:

	Tons	Guns
Lawrence	260	20
Niagara	260	20
Caledonia	85	3
Ariel	60	4
Somers	65	2
Scorpion	60	2

Porcupine	50	1
Tigress	50	1
Trippe	50	1

Captain Robert H. Barclay RN commanded the British fleet consisting of:

	Tons	Guns
Detroit	300	19
Queen Charlotte	200	17
Lady Prevost	96	13
General Hunter	75	10
Little Belt	60	3
Chippewa	35	1

It is worth noting that, from the time that war was declared, only one major fighting vessel was built at Fort Malden. This vessel was the *Detroit*. The Americans, on the other hand, had built two large brigs, and four gunboats at Presque Isle, and had seven small ships. The British had four ships, of which one, the *General Hunter*, was unfit for use as early as 1811. Undoubtedly, the activity in the yard at Presque Isle far surpassed that at Fort Malden, and this was largely due to the availability of skilled workers, armaments and all supplies being far superior for the Americans. Possibly there was also a difference in the standards to which the ships were built in the two yards. Yet how could the *Detroit* withstand such a battering during the battle? It appears she was built in the fashion of the Admiralty dockyards with frames only a few inches apart, thus making virtually a wooden wall, some 18 inches or more thick. The American ships were more lightly framed. This follows Noah Brown's dictum as quoted earlier in the section on shipbuilding.

The book, *Naval Monument*, by the American A. Bowen, although blatantly propagandistic and written during the war in a style that is reminiscent of a recruitment effort, contains a copy of a letter of September 13 from Commodore Perry to the secretary of

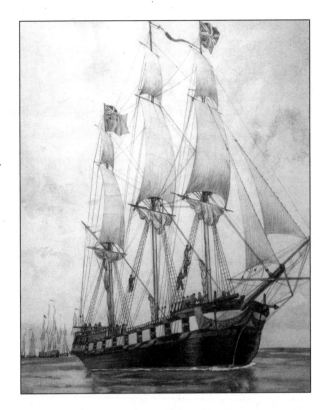

Captain Robert H. Barclay's flagship, the Detroit, *built at Fort Malden in 1813, was lost in the Battle of Lake Erie a mere few weeks after launching. C.H.J. Snider, artist.* Courtesy of TRL, T15242.

the Navy. It states, in part, "The *Detroit* is a remarkably fine ship, sails well, and is very strongly built."[1] He also comments on the superior qualities of the *Queen Charlotte* and the *Lady Prevost*. Bowen also prints a letter from someone described as "a naval officer", written and dated at Erie, October 7, 1813, "Our short guns lodged their shot in the bulwarks of the *Detroit*, where a number of them now remain. Her bulwarks however, are vastly superior to ours, being of oak and very thick."[2] The officer writes of shot going "quite through" the walls of the *Lawrence*.

Furthermore, it was Admiralty custom to protect those operating the guns and working the ship on the main deck of its men-of-war with heavy, shoulder-high bulwarks that were quite effective in warding off many injuries. The smaller vessels, or converted merchantmen, would not normally offer this protection, and such security from death or injury does not appear to have been offered on the American vessels on Lake Erie.

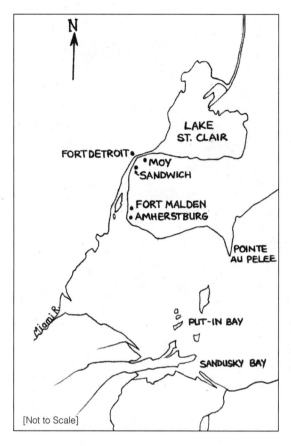

Map of the western part of Lake Erie and the Detroit River. Sketch by Heidi Hoffman.

The naval leaders on both sides proved to be heroes worth remembering and honouring. The same goes for most of the men. The only exception of note was Lieutenant Jesse Elliott, commander of the *USS Niagara*, who all during the battle kept his brig out of range of the British ships until the fighting was almost over. He was roundly accused of "cowardice" and caused quite a scandal at the time. However, when Perry's *Lawrence* had been virtually demolished by the guns of the *Detroit*, Perry abandoned his ship and took over command of the *Niagara*. Thus, he was able to bring a fresh vessel into the fray. It became the deciding factor.

One amazing feature of the battle, which took place at Put-in-Bay among some islands in Lake Erie, is how well the untrained soldiers and sailors performed. Both sides had good reason to complain about the skills of the men sent to operate their ships. Perry's people

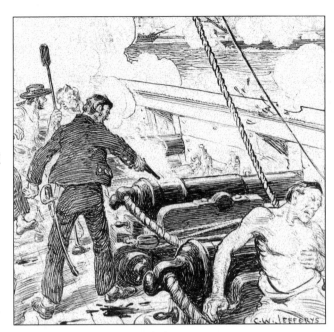

Some of the cannon on the Detroit *had to be fired by igniting the powder with a pistol shot. This requirement would certainly slow down the firing rate. Sketch by C.W. Jefferys.* Courtesy of Library and Archives Canada, C73575.

also suffered from fever up to the day of battle. Barclay had more landsmen than navy men on the *Detroit*. They did not "know the ropes," they had never fired a cannon before, partly because there was insufficient gunpowder with which to practise. Also, they had to fight with six different sizes of guns, which meant six different sizes of balls and powder cartridges. Furthermore, some of the guns did not have flintlocks that worked. They had to be touched off by firing pistols at the vents. Historian Robert Malcolmson, who did a great deal of research on the subject, determined that Barclay's crew totalled 434, of which 188 were from the Royal Navy, 146 were soldiers from the 41st Regiment, 98 were from the Newfoundlanders (a regiment of British soldiers from Newfoundland) and there were two unidentified Native warriors. It is interesting to note, though unexplained, that the *Little Belt* and the *Chippewa* were manned by teenagers.[3]

This lack of skilled seamen probably contributed to the collision of the *Detroit* and *Queen Charlotte* during the battle. It scarcely could have helped Barclay's efforts when two of his own ships collided, but in the heat of a major battle, even the best of trained men could not always prevent such an accident. The tonnage of the ships, and their armaments has been a matter of dispute among writers since the day of the battle. The range of discussion over the battle is not the issue of this work, other than to point out that Barclay on the *Detroit* had more long guns, taken from the fort at Malden, permitting him to do more damage from a greater distance, which contributed to the destruction of the *Lawrence*. Perry's guns were carronades, capable of firing a much heavier broadside than Barclay's long guns but with a shorter range. Once the ships came closer together, there was really very little hope for the *Detroit*.

Without distracting in any way from the leadership skills or fighting qualities of the men on either side, it is evident that the better "tools" won the battle. The ships that were built at Presque Isle were not superior to those built at Fort Malden, but were more in number and much better armed. For this the blame falls, not on the builders but on those whose job it was to provide the materials, guns and skilled men to equip Barclay's fleet. As noted earlier, the cannon, which had been shipped from England months previously and hauled overland from Quebec, had been captured by the Americans when they occupied York in April 1813. It is my speculation that Barclay lost the battle primarily because the guns he needed had been lost to the Americans at York. The guns he was able to scramble together were a real mixture, some even being field artillery from Fort Malden.

Following the Battle of Fort Erie, affairs became very quiet on the Upper Lakes. All the major players had left the stage. The shipyard at Presque Isle was essentially closed down, a great change from all the hustle and bustle earlier in the year. The yard at Fort Malden had been burned down, and, for all intents and purposes, was totally destroyed.

It seemed that the Americans controlled the Upper Lakes. Or did they? On December 19, 1813, the British burned Buffalo, and at Black Rock they burned two of Perry's ships, the *Ariel* and the *Trippe* and captured the *Little Belt*. On August 1, 1814, two British vessels, the *Charwell*, under Lieutenant Alex Dobbs, and the *Netley* under the command of Copeland Radcliffe, were anchored in the Niagara River near Queenston when they learned that the Americans had positioned three armed schooners in the entrance to the river

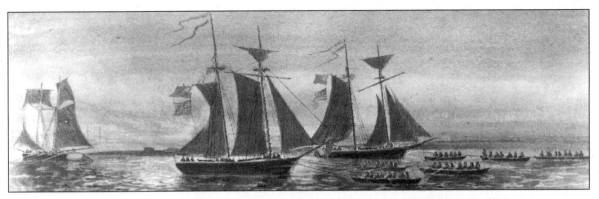

The capture of the USN Somers *(centre foreground) and the* USN Ohio *(to the left), just off the entrance to the Niagara River on August 12, 1814. C.J.H. Snider, artist.* Courtesy of TRL, JRR 1163.

between Fort Erie and Buffalo. These were the *Ohio* (60 tons), the *Somers* (99 tons) and the *Porcupine* (83 tons). All three had been part of Perry's fleet in the Battle of Lake Erie.

Dobbs and Radcliffe took it into their heads to try to cut out these vessels and to capture them. The British had no ships available on Lake Erie to play a part, so the captain's gig from the *Charwell* was carried on the shoulders of the sailors from Queenston to Lake Erie. It took two nights of heavy marching, for they did not want to expose themselves by day, to reach Lake Erie with the heavy 20-foot gig. Near the mouth of Frenchman's Creek on the Niagara, some three or four miles below Lake Erie, they found five flat-bottomed bateaux hauled up on the bank. They carried these as well, to a launching spot some five miles upstream from Fort Erie.

At dawn on August 12, the British again had a little fleet on Lake Erie – one gig and five bateaux. Just after midnight that night, they drifted down on the three schooners. After a fight of short duration, perhaps 15 to 30 minutes, they captured the *Ohio* and the *Somers* with few casualties. However, the *Porcupine* managed to escape.

The British had started building two schooners at the old shipyard at Chippawa, near Navy Island, a few miles above the Falls in the Niagara River, but they were not completed in time to take part in the war. These vessels were the *Tecumseth* and the *Newash*, launched on

August 15, 1815, and used on the Upper Lakes until 1832 when they sank at Penetang, in disrepair at the end of their service. Their work included transport of British troops and goods, both military and civilian during this period. They also did customs patrol to prevent smuggling and sought out deserters, occasioning a few disputes with the American authorities. Barry Gough, in *Fighting Sail on Lake Huron and Georgian Bay*, offers some very engaging details regarding the history and the evolution of the naval centre at Penetanguishine.

In August 1814, the British had 24 bateaux in use above the Falls. They continued to hold Fort Mackinac until after peace was declared though there were problems keeping it supplied.

> Through winter's snow, through summer's heat, No more the sentry walks his beat.
> No morning guard-mounts now reveal
> The scarlet dress, the glancing steel; No more at rise and set of sun,
> Is heard the morn and evening gun, Of those who made the scene so fair, And lent the place its martial air, Full many sleep – their graves are green, The drooping willows o'er them lean,
> And mould'ring headstones scarcely tell of name, or birth-place loved so well; No rolling drum, no stirring fife,
> Can ever call them back to life, Till sounds the final reveille – In every land, on every sea
> That wakes all; for the grand review. Whose lights went out at Death's tattoo.[4]

What happened to Barclay's *HMS Detroit* after the battle? She remained at Put-in-Bay through the winter of 1813–14, along with the hulks of Perry's *USS Lawrence* and the *HMS Queen Charlotte*. In 1814, all three vessels were taken to Erie and anchored in Misery Bay, part of the harbour there. Masts were taken out and presumably the vessels were covered to protect them from the weather. They were later stripped of everything of value and scuttled in the anchorage to preserve them along with the *Niagara*. It seems that different people bought them at different times, but never took possession. However, at what became the final sale in 1837, the *Detroit* was raised and repaired and put into service as was the *Queen Charlotte*. The *Lawrence* was raised in 1874, and the *Niagara* in 1913. It is possible that timbers were probably salvaged from the others and, if so, would have been used in construction.

Ultimately, the *Detroit* and the *Queen Charlotte* were refitted as merchantmen and put into service, but they did not last long. By 1841 the *Detroit* had become a derelict yet again, and was floated down the Niagara River with the idea of sending her over the Falls as an entertainment event. She did not surrender willingly. She grounded in the rapids above the Falls and over a period of some weeks, she gradually broke up and went over in pieces. Thus ended the brave ship *Detroit*.

CHAPTER 11

Disaffection

IN THE YEARS JUST PRECEDING THE WAR, the north shores of the St. Lawrence, Lake Ontario and Lake Erie were much more settled than the south shores. At this time, Canadian farmers in Upper Canada exported much produce to the United States. The Thames Valley area of southwestern Upper Canada was the breadbasket of the Great Lakes Basin. When the country was invaded following the Battle of Lake Erie in 1813, many farms were laid waste and, even worse, the flour mills were destroyed by the invaders.

Similarly, the flour mills at Port Dover, Port Ryerse, Port Talbot and other villages were destroyed in raids. Some writers suggest that much of this destruction was carried out by disaffected Canadians along with Americans who had immigrated into Upper Canada as settlers in the years just before the war. As a result, farm produce, particularly flour and meat, fell into very short supply in Upper Canada. At times, the military forces were placed on short rations and food had to be imported from Britain. The situation was exacerbated by the requirement that the government provide food for the Native allies – the men, their wives and their children.

Whether from sympathy for the British cause, or more likely, to take advantage of the situation and because they could get higher prices for their produce in Canada than in the United States, American farmers in Vermont and New York supplied huge quantities of cattle to the British forces. Similarly, the farmers south of Lake Erie supplied quantities of flour. However, there were also many cases when flour was shipped from Canada to American towns that were also suffering a shortage. Undoubtedly, these undertakings were treasonable acts, but, in some cases, the authorities were participating in the illicit deals themselves. Historic records do not show that any action was taken against the parties by either government.

Canada was faced with a considerable problem. There was a great suspicion of disaffection, a swelling of discontentedness directed against the political structures that became viewed as disloyalty. General Isaac Brock reported, "The population, believe me, are a bad lot."[1] There were cases of desertion to the enemy from the Canadian militia, particularly around Amherstburg when the Americans invaded, and also on the Niagara frontier. More seriously, there were many cases of recruiting and the coercion of otherwise loyal, or at least neutral, citizens into open disaffection.

It was noted earlier that when the Americans captured York in the spring of 1813, one of the casualties was the burning of the Parliament Houses. Some writers have suggested that this was an act of vandalism on the part of some American soldiers. Investigation does not support this opinion, but rather indicates that the more likely villains were American settlers from the countryside around York, some of whom had the idea that they would be better off if America won the war and added the new State of Canada to their nation.

Following the American War of Independence, there was a great influx of settlers from America. Tens of thousands of United Empire Loyalists, who maintained loyalty to the Crown of Great Britain, immigrated to Upper Canada. History records that they became loyal and, for the most part, prosperous citizens who were a great asset to the young country. Soon, another class of immigrants entered in very large numbers. These were migrants from America

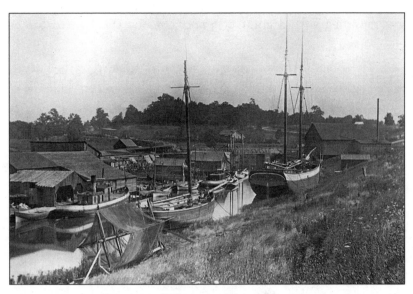

After the hamlet of Dover Mills on Lake Erie was razed by the Americans in the War of 1812, reconstruction took place closer to the mouth of the Lynn River, where a harbour had been in use since the early 1800s. Harbour improvements made the new Port Dover a principal Lake Erie port with ship-yards, tanneries and Andrew Thompson's woollen mill that contributed substantially to local economic growth. Shown here in this photo, c.1890, are the sloop Viking *(left) and the schooner* Erie Stewart *in the Lynn River. Both these vessels were built locally in the 1870s. There also are a number of fishing boats – both steam and sail – along the creek and a net-drying reel in the foreground.* Courtesy of the Port Dover Harbour Museum.

who had no loyalty to the president but certainly equally no allegiance to the Crown. They received most of the blame for vandalism, arson and incitement to traitorous acts.

When the Americans held Fort George at Newark in 1814, some 120 or so traitors formed a local corps of refugees known as the Canadian Volunteers and became part of the American garrison at Fort George. Some writers have claimed that these voluntaries were responsible for burning the town of Newark. Since they were under the command of the American forces, the Americans were generally blamed for this act of vandalism against a defenceless town. The same Canadian Volunteers formed part of the invasion force that captured Fort Erie in July 1814. The leader of this corps, one Abraham Markle, was rewarded with a grant of 3,000 acres by the United States government.

The group from Amherstburg, who had defected to the enemy, raided settlements in Middlesex and Oxford counties, kidnapped militia at Delaware, at Oxford and at Port Talbot and along the Talbot Road, burning houses and mills, destroying crops and killing livestock. After the peace treaty was ratified, some of the brigands tried to re-enter Canada as immigrant settlers. A list of 336 names of such outlaws was drawn up but probably there were many more. Congress rewarded them for their services to the American cause. One writer indicates that many were recruited to these acts of treason by the incentive of such rewards.

Apart from having their property confiscated, most of the offenders went unpunished. But not all were excused. In December 1813, a group of American marauders were captured in a house near Chatham. Among them were 15 residents of Upper Canada. Those from the United States were held as prisoners of war. They were not traitors. The others were held for trial under a charge of treason. Four more were arrested and added to the list. Others, not captured, were tried in absentia, in order that they might be outlawed.

In May and June, a trial took place at Ancaster. A large number of the 19 men were determined to have arrived from the United States only a year or two before the war broke out. Were they purposely embedded, or had they immigrated into Canada of their own volition, foreseeing that, from that position, they could benefit the American side? The records do not answer this question.

To make a long and unpleasant story short, four of the 19 were acquitted, 15 were found guilty, were convicted and condemned to be hanged. On June 20, 1814, eight were executed by hanging. The other seven were transported to Kingston to the prison there, from which four escaped, though three were recaptured. Three died of typhus in prison and the others were pardoned on the condition that they leave Upper Canada for life. Of those tried in absentia, thirty were judged to be outlaws and their property was confiscated by the Crown. The American government, having promised to reward the Canadian traitors, made land grants to some of these outlaws who returned to the United Sates.

It must be made clear that there was no case reported of disaffection by any immigrant who came to Canada as a direct result of the American War of Independence. The United Empire Loyalists showed their loyalty to the Crown at every opportunity. There appears to have been a considerable number of more recent homesteaders who were not so loyal. The challenges of disaffection were trying indeed.

In the words of John Lord O'Brian, an American anti-trust lawyer, now deceased, "There is something peculiarly sinister and insidious in even a charge of disloyalty. Such a charge all too frequently places a strain on the reputation of an individual which is indelible and lasting, regardless of the complete innocence later proved."

CHAPTER 12

Negotiations for Peace

ALTHOUGH NOT REALLY CONCERNED with the story of sail on the Great Lakes, a brief outline of the negotiations to a long and lasting peace settlement on the world's longest undefended border is of interest here.

Quite early in the war, in May 1813, President James Madison sent envoys to Europe to start negotiations for peace. Napoleon had been defeated in Moscow and there was the possibility of a French defeat in Europe. As has already been noted, this accomplishment would release large British armies and greater naval forces for service in North America.

John Quincy Adams, Henry Clay and three others were immediately appointed to become peace commissioners on behalf of the United States and negotiations commenced. Meanwhile the war would continue. The American delegation to the peace negotiations had been directed to demand that the Royal Navy put an end to its practice of impressing sailors. They were to renegotiate the matters of naval blockades and maritime rights, and to try to secure the secession of the two Canadas to the United States.[1]

The five American commissioners soon realized how empty-headed these instructions were. It was clear that America, in 1814, would have difficulty compelling Britain to agree to anything, other than the status quo, ante bellum. The American delegation eventually received more sensible instructions, permitting them to modify their stand in the negotiations for peace. Internally the United States was having economic difficulty. Trade was at a standstill. Banks were failing and paper money was being heavily discounted. Only a fraction of the federal government's latest war loan was subscribed. The regular army was declining in strength because there were not enough recruits to make good its wastage. Worst of all, there was a growing movement in New England for secession from the United States and the creation of its own federation.

Britain pressed for "restoration to the Indian nations of all their rights, privileges and territories, which they had enjoyed in the year 1811." The American negotiators took the stance that the Natives were "merely dwellers in the United States," however, agreement was reached to restore them to the rights enjoyed before 1811. However, as Alfred Mahan records, "In the light of subsequent history it is difficult to see how they could have agreed to it in good faith.... From July to October 1815, the United States signed fifteen treaties with diverse Indian tribes guaranteeing each their status as of 1811. But in none of these did it return one acre of land."[2]

The British soon came to the realization that they were powerless to enforce the position of restoration to the First Nations People involved. However, they did obtain an agreement that both parties "would use their best endeavours to promote the entire abolition of the slave trade." In subsequent years, the American government insisted that Britain either return slaves (who had sought freedom in Canada) to their previous owners or pay for them. Britain refused to return the African Americans, for they would be enslaved again. In 1827, Britain paid £250,000 in full settlement for some 3,600 slaves.

War costs in both countries were extremely high. In the United States, they were estimated at $105 million. For Britain it is difficult to arrive at a figure, but it is believed to be a much higher amount than this. Towards the end of the negotiations it appeared that war

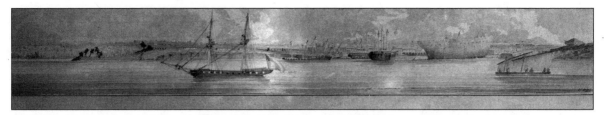

Sacket's Harbor, 1815, after peace was declared. The New Orleans *can be seen in the stocks. Many vessels have already had their yards removed. The brig* Jones, *shown in the foreground, is still rigged. E.E. Vidal, artist.* Courtesy of the Massey Library, Royal Military College, Kingston, Ontario.

was about to break out again in Europe. Consequently, Britain made concessions that otherwise might have required further prolonging the war. She had already been at war for 21 years and her people were tired of the high taxes needed to support war efforts.

The negotiators finally reached an agreement acceptable to both parties and the Treaty of Ghent was signed on Christmas Eve 1814. In brief, all conquests were to be returned; the boundary was to be defined by subsequent international commissions. Ironically, nowhere in the treaty was there any reference to blockades or impressments, the stated reasons given by the United States for the declaration of war in the first place. Neither country won an acre of extra territory. Neither side won the war. John Jacob Astor was the only winner, for he ended up with a virtual monopoly of the fur trade in the areas where he was operating. The North West Company and the Hudson's Bay Company restricted their activities to north of the new border.

The United States emerged from the war with a "heightened national feeling," according to Mahan. "They are more American. They feel and act more as a nation." During the war American interests had expanded manufacturing equal to what would have been expected only after ten decades of peace."[3] This was partly due to the blockade and partly to meet the urgent demands of the military. In Canada, a great feeling of patriotism had emerged. Hostility and distrust of the United States remained very real in both England and in British North America for many years afterwards.

Herbert Agar, writing in 1950 in *The Price of Union*, notes, "Perhaps it is well that no one told America that her new freedom depended not on the Treaty of Ghent, but on the Treaty of Fontainebleau, which had been signed on May 30, 1814, after Napoleon's abdication. It was not the little war against England, which won for America the blessing of being left alone; it was the enormous war against Europe's conqueror. With Napoleon beaten, and England supreme at sea, the world was to know relative peace for one hundred years; and within that peace the United States was safe, and grew strong."[4]

Looking back from this moment, the war is remembered by very few, other than historians. The Americans think of it primarily as a naval war in which "Britain's pride was humbled by the American upstart." They prefer to forget that they accomplished none of the purposes for which they declared war. The Canadians think of it with pride as a war of defence in which their brave forefathers turned back the massed might of the United States, whereas it was the professional British soldier and the seaman with the help of the Natives, who deserved most of the credit. The British do not even remember it happened.

CHAPTER 13

The Saga of the *Nancy*

WHEN FORT MACKINAC FELL TO THE BRITISH IN 1812, President Madison is reported to have commented, "We have just learned that the important post of Michilimackinac has fallen into the hands of the enemies, but from what cause remains to be known." It is not reported what remarks he offered when he learned of the defeat of the American forces that were sent to recapture the fort in the summer of 1814.

Commander Arthur Sinclair USN had taken command of the American navy in the Upper Lakes in the spring of 1814. He was instructed, along with Major George Croghan, to retake the fort. In June, he set out to do so, taking the *Niagara*, the *Hunter*, the *Caledonia* and the schooners, the *Tigress* and the *Scorpion*. The ships were manned by more than five hundred seamen and marines and were transporting nearly one thousand soldiers. Obviously the cabinet in Washington considered this endeavour to be a very important project. As long as the British held the fort, they controlled the Upper Lakes and the fur trade. This site was a key trading post for Astor's fur business and the British had captured a quantity of furs belonging to him when they took the island in 1812. Astor had made large loans to the American government in support of the war and Washington felt

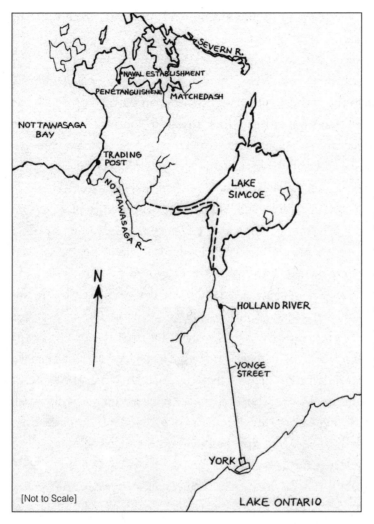

Sketch map of the overland route from York to Lake Simcoe, then via the Nottawasaga River to Nottawasaga Bay and on to the naval establishment at Penetanguishene and to Matchedash. Map by Heidi Hoffman.

obligated to try to recover his property. When Sinclair arrived at Mackinac, he was surprised to find Astor's agents had arrived ahead of him and were busy negotiating the return of the furs.

In charge of the fort was Lieutenant-Colonel Robert McDouall of the Glengarry Light Infantry, who had served under Sir James Yeo at Kingston, and is also reported to have fought at the Battle of Sacket's Harbor on May 29, 1813. He had only assumed command in May. He marched up Yonge Street to Lake Simcoe, crossed the lake on the ice in February, then portaged to the Nottawasaga River and arranged for bateaux to be built there. He had brought shipwrights to Mackinac with him for that purpose. In addition, McDouall was accompanied by 21 seamen, 11 artillerymen and two companies of soldiers from the Royal Newfoundland Regiment. On April 19, he started down the river with 30 bateaux, heavily laden with provisions and military stores. On the 25th, he set out across Georgian Bay for Fort Mackinac in boisterous spring weather. It took 19 days in "open and deeply laden bateaux across the expanse of Lake Huron covered with immense fields of ice and agitated by violent gales of wind."[1] He arrived without loss of man or supplies, though one bateaux was wrecked.

At Mackinac, McDouall had only one transport to bring in supplies and move troops. This was the *Nancy*, the only one of Robert Barclay's vessels to escape the Battle of Lake Erie. Actually, she was still privately owned at the time but employed by Barclay to carry men and supplies to faraway forts. On the day of the battle she was going about her regular transport duties on Lake Huron and was unaware of the American victory until she tried to put in at Moy House, Sandwich, on October 13, 1813. She headed back up the lake and spent the winter at the North West Company's post at St. Mary's (now Sault Ste. Marie) where repairs were made and new sails fitted. The following spring she brought two loads of supplies from Matchedash to Fort Mackinac and was on her way back for a third when the American fleet entered the lake.

In the spring of 1814, the private transport vessel, the *Nancy*, owned by the North West Company, was taken over by the Royal Navy and became the *HMS Nancy*. Alexander Mackintosh stayed on as sailing master. Lieutenant Miller Worsley RN was assigned by Commodore Yeo to command the British vessels on Lake Huron, the *HMS Nancy* (from hereafter the ship will simply be referred to as *Nancy*) and the *Mink*. Worsley was a young, energetic officer who had spent several years in the Navy, fought at Trafalgar, and served on a number of vessels in the Lake Ontario fleet.

The Americans arrived in Lake Huron on July 12, but instead of going straight to Fort Mackinac, they changed course for Matchedash Bay where Commander Sinclair had been told the British were storing large quantities of supplies and were building gunboats. Unable to

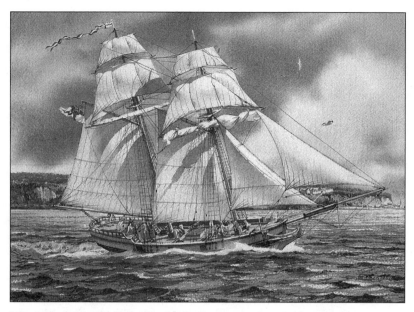

The Nancy Under Sail. *Charles L. Peterson, artist. Built at Detroit in 1789, she sailed lakes Huron and Erie as armed transport until destroyed by fire in the Nottawasaga River in 1814. Her remains can be seen at Nancy Island Historic Site, Wasaga Beach Provincial Park, Wasaga Beach, Ontario.*

find Matchedash without charts or a pilot familiar with the area, they next headed for Fort St. Joseph on St. Joseph Island, about ten miles south of St. Mary's. They looted and burned what was left of the fort and were successful in capturing the North West Company transport, *Mink*, which was heading for St. Mary's with supplies for the post. Learning that the *Perseverance*, another company vessel, was waiting for the *Mink* before proceeding west on Lake Superior to Fort William, Sinclair sent the *Scorpion* ahead to try to capture her. After plundering the strategic fur trading post at St. Mary's, the Americans burned and destroyed storehouses, a sawmill and garden plots. Even grain supplies and the horses in the stable were burned. They also destroyed the 2580-foot timber canal and towpath built by the fur company to bypass the rapids at St. Mary's.

Proceeding above the rapids, the Americans found the *Perseverance* already on fire. She was captured, but, in an attempt to bring her down the treacherous river into Lake Huron, "she bilged...but we succeeded in running her ashore below the rapids before she filled, and we burned her."[2]

The Americans now had control of Lake Superior, and, had it not been for the force at Fort Mackinac, they would have pushed on to wipe out the British fur trade by attacking Fort William. Interestingly, they had missed by only two days the forty-seven Company boats laden with furs valued to a million dollars that had slipped through the canal, en route from Fort William to Montreal via the French River. The American fleet then proceeded to Mackinac, where they arrived on July 26. Both a naval attack and an attempt to land and take the place were unsuccessful. The army suffered considerable losses and withdrew.

Major Croghan had learned of the *Nancy* and that she had been dispatched to the Nottawasaga River for another load of supplies. He was determined to capture or to destroy her. The odds should have been in their favour: six ships and some 1,400 men against one small transport, armed with three guns and with only a handful of men. Croghan had not been able to capture the fort with all his ships, men and munitions. Perhaps he could starve them out. Certainly the fort needed a continuous supply of arms and provisions, not only for the military, but also for the hundreds of Native warriors and their families. Keeping them satisfied was deemed essential, for fear they might otherwise disappear, or even worse, join the enemy forces.

Fortunately for the *Nancy*, when the American fleet appeared, McDouall was able to send a warning to her. Robert Livingston, an official of the Indian Department, had volunteered to deliver the message, and had set off by canoe.

About the middle of July, Lieutenant Miller Worsley with a small detachment of seamen, had arrived at the mouth of the Nottawasaga River. There he awaited the arrival of the *Nancy*, suffering much discomfort from bad weather and being pestered by swarms of mosquitoes. When the *Nancy* reached her destination, she was loaded with 300 barrels of flour, salt pork, and other provisions along with military stores. On August 1, she was ready to set sail back to Mackinac when Livingston arrived with the news that the American fleet was nearby in the lake. The *Nancy* was towed about two miles up the Nottawasaga River where she was hidden from view from offshore. A log blockhouse was quickly erected and her guns transferred into it. On August 13, the American fleet, comprised of the *Niagara*, *Scorpion* and *Tigress*, arrived. The other vessels had been sent back to Erie.

Worsley had only 21 seamen, one midshipman, 21 Natives, and nine French-Canadian boatmen. Livingston was dispatched overland to York to seek more troops for defence of the *Nancy*. However, the British forces were engaged in attacking Fort Erie in an attempt to recapture the fort back from the Americans, so a messenger was also sent on to Fort Erie. Livingston returned to Wasaga, and although no reinforcements were believed to be forthcoming, he was able to round up an additional 23 Indians to serve.

Croghan did not know the *Nancy* was hidden upriver, but he ordered a contingent of troops ashore to select a campsite, as he was prepared to wait out the arrival of the schooner. His men discovered the *Nancy's* masts glinting through the trees back alongside the river. Next morning, Commander Sinclair anchored near the shore and opened fire, but with little effect, since not being able to see the schooner and the blockhouse from offshore made it difficult to direct the fire. He then moved men to the beaches with howitzers, and was able to place them within a few hundred yards of the *Nancy*. However, Worsley was determined that the *Nancy* would not fall into enemy hands. He spiked the guns at the blockhouse and prepared to blow up the vessel when a lucky shot destroyed the blockhouse and, at the same time, ignited the explosives on the *Nancy*. She burned to the waterline and sank in the river.

Sinclair investigated the wreck, removed the guns from the blockhouse and felled trees across the mouth of the river to prevent its further use. He then withdrew to Erie with the *Niagara*, where he learned of the loss of the *Somers* and the *Ohio* to the British at Fort Erie. He left Lieutenant Daniel Turner in command of the *Scorpion* and the *Tigress* to maintain a blockade of the Nottawasaga for as long as weather permitted. He authorized Turner to patrol intermittently to the north between St. Joseph and the French River, and warned him to be cautious and to prevent any possibility of his ships being boarded. If they were successful in preventing supplies from reaching Fort Mackinac until October, the British surely would be starved out during the winter. A brigade of boats bringing supplies from Montreal received warning about the American blockade while they were still in the French River. They were able to turn back to safety.

Worsley was left with a sunken and useless schooner, but he had two bateaux and Livingston's large canoe, plus almost 100 barrels of provisions that had survived the attack. He managed to get out of the river and elude the blockade on the night of August 18, and headed up through the Thirty Thousand Islands and the North Channel towards Fort Mackinac. Near St. Joseph, after rowing 360 miles, he discovered the two schooners that had been blockading the Nottawasaga, cruising among the islands. He promptly hid his two bateaux in a secluded bay, and, under cover of darkness, and with all his men in Livingston's canoe, he was able to pass by the Americans unobserved. On September 1, 1814 at sunset, they reached the safety of Fort Mackinac.

He quickly got permission from McDouall to try to capture the schooners and next day set out with four large bateaux and some 70 soldiers and seamen. Two hundred Natives in 19 canoes accompanied them, but they took little part in the events to follow. At dusk on September 2, the force arrived at Detour Passage between the upper peninsula of Michigan and Drummond Island where the St. Mary's River empties into Lake Huron. The men were landed there and the boats carefully hidden. Next day, Worsley and Livingston reconnoitred ahead by canoe and discovered one of the schooners, the *Tigress*, at anchor about six miles away. At dusk that day, the whole force re-embarked, and rowed as quietly as possible towards the enemy. The Natives were instructed to remain behind, but three of the principal chiefs were taken into the boats thus making a total force of ninety-two. Quietly, the four bateaux crept up on the schooner and boarded her with little warning. A brief fight ensued before she was captured. The prisoners were put under guard and sent to Michilimackinac by boat, and Livingston was sent out to find the *Scorpion*. During the night of September 5, three days later, they spotted the ship anchored within five miles of the *Tigress*, quite unaware of what had transpired. At daybreak, next morning, the *Tigress* sailed slowly down to her, under jib and foresail, and some dozen yards away fired the twenty-four pounder into her hull, then quickly ran alongside and grappled her. With practically no resistance, the *Scorpion* was captured.

Participating in this action was Lieutenant David Wingfield, remembered by present-day sailors through the name of a small harbour of refuge at the tip of Bruce Peninsula, named Wingfield Basin. He also left us a detailed journal. A person is permitted to include, in his private journal, or exclude, items as he sees fit! And Wingfield was no exception. He neglected to mention in his writings that, when bringing the *HMS Surprise* (ex *Scorpion*) into the Penetanguishene harbour after a survey expedition, he ran her across a shoal and broke the lower pintle, part of the rudder fittings. Some iron salvaged from the *Nancy* was used for the repairs.

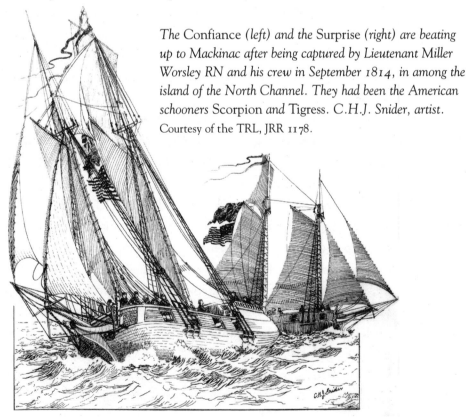

The Confiance *(left) and the* Surprise *(right) are beating up to Mackinac after being captured by Lieutenant Miller Worsley RN and his crew in September 1814, in among the island of the North Channel. They had been the American schooners* Scorpion *and* Tigress. *C.H.J. Snider, artist.* Courtesy of the TRL, JRR 1178.

Now, with the capture of both the *Tigress* and the *Scorpion*, McDouall had relatively new schooners to replace the *Nancy* and keep the fort supplied. The Americans made no further attempt to attack Fort Mackinac, but what they had been unable to do by force of arms or by blockade, they succeeded in doing at the peace table.

While the *Scorpion* was renamed the *Surprise*, the *Tigress* became the *Confiance*. They would serve the British for many years. The *Confiance*, under the command of Worsley, was used in lake-survey duty with Captain William Fitzwilliam Owen RN after whom Owen's Sound and ultimately the town of Owen Sound were named, and who became a world-famous explorer and surveyor of the African continent. In 1817, both vessels were reassigned to the mouth of the Grand River (present-day Dunnville, Ontario) to serve all of lakes Erie and Huron, including Penetanguishene adjacent to Georgian Bay. The *Confiance* carried David Thompson, the famous mapmaker and explorer, during his work with the International Boundary Commission.

Both vessels were back at the Grand River in 1821, and again in 1831, when they were "…to be broken up and their names erased from the lists of the Royal Navy."[3] It appears that they ended their days on Lake Erie where the American, Daniel Dobbins had built them at Presque Isle in December 1812.

The *Nancy* was first built for the firm of Forsyth, Richardson and Company, Montreal fur merchants, at the Ship Yard Tract, which later became Woodmere Cemetery along the Rouge River, six miles or so south of Fort Detroit. John Richardson, one of the firm's partners, went to Detroit to keep an eye on the work. "The schooner," he wrote on September 23, 1789, "will be a perfect masterpiece of workmanship and beauty. The expense to us will be great, but there will be the satisfaction of her being strong and very durable. Her floor timbers, keel, keelson, stem and lower futtock are oak. The transom, stern post, upper futtocks, top timbers, beams and knees are all red cedar. She will carry 350 barrels."[4]

He arranged for a figurehead, "…a lady dressed in the present fashion with a hat and feather"[5] to be carved by Skelling of New York. The *Nancy* was launched on September 24, 1789, "…a most

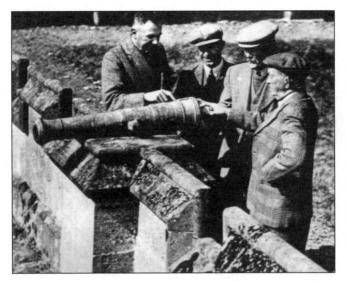

Chief Lachlan Mackintosh of Mackintosh, shows friends one of the Nancy's *guns at Moy Hall, County of Inverness, Scotland, photo not dated. The guns were imported into Scotland in 1836.* Courtesy of the Ontario Department of Tourism, now Ministry of Tourism.

beautiful and substantial vessel."[6] The next spring, she started her work of carrying cargo, supplies and furs all over Lake Erie and to Sault Ste. Marie and Fort Mackinac.

During her building, the yard was visited from time to time by Alexander Mackintosh, a partner in the North West Company at Moy, (at Sandwich, now Windsor) and by "wee Alec," his three-year-old nephew who enjoyed sailing adze chips in the puddles and even in the river. Alexander Mackintosh became captain of the *Nancy* around 1800 when the NWC acquired her and remained her captain throughout the war. He stayed in Canada at Moy House until 1827, then returned to Scotland where he died in 1833.

According to Snider, the *Nancy* was 58 feet from stem to stern post, perhaps 65 feet on deck, by no means a large boat. In 1793, she was sold to the George Leith Company, and described as being of 67 tons burthen. At the outbreak of the war she was lying at the North West Company base at Moy House. Lieutenant-Colonel St. George took her into the Provincial Marine as an armed transport. While in service for the fur-trading companies she had been armed with two small brass cannon, but these were taken out of her when she was taken over at Moy. Undoubtedly, she was re-armed, but no record of what guns she carried could be found.

As an interesting aside, in 1836, Alexander Mackintosh of Mackintosh, Chief of Clan Chattan, imported into Scotland two brass cannon, two pounders, formerly of the *Nancy*, and they are now mounted on a wall outside Moy Hall at Inverness, Scotland. This fact has been confirmed to me in direct communication with Lachlan Mackintosh of Mackintosh.

The average life of a ship in those years, with reasonable maintenance, was ten years. The *Nancy* served 23 years in the fur trade and an additional two years as a transport for the Provincial Marine. In the trade, she carried supplies to all the outposts on the Upper Lakes and brought back furs and local produce.

One of the principal merchants of Detroit at the time was John Askin, who had lived there while it was British, but moved to Canada in 1802, locating at Strabane, now Walkerville. He had a large family whose members settled in various spots around the lakes, and wrote back and forth, creating a great many letters, most of which have been retained. It is fascinating to read this family correspondence, and to learn from it, some of the cargo carried by the *Nancy*.

As well as produce, corn, flour, whisky, salt, sugar, furs, clothing and such, there were included "apple trees in tubs," barrels of apples and barrels of cider. In one case, a complaint was made that the "working of the vessel increases the fermentation of the cyder and very often not only lessens the Quantity but injures the Quality."

On one occasion, daughter Archange requests that her father send her a "cariole" (a light buggy with awning) and son John, at St. Joseph on November 11, 1809, sends his father a barrel of whitefish and two extras for friends, and adds, "I should be happy to get a Dozen or less of Apple Tree plants the size of half an inch in diameter or more. The roots may be put in a small keg pressed together and filled with earth and the limbs twisted in straw to prevent their receiving any injury."

The father writes back and requests he send a "bark of sugar, abt 30 lb. wt." Father promises to send an "American ox" from Sandwich and the "R. Tranche" (the Thames), also breeding sows and geese. His mother wants a good buffalo skin and thanks him for the "Cranberry Confiture." John, in Mackinac, replying to his father, promises to send a "moccock" and adds, "...the Mich. and S.W. Fur Co. ... have now on board the Caledonia from 12 to 15,000 pounds of sugar for McIntosh." Agricultural implements, a ploughshare and irons, are discussed in a letter of 1810. John asked his father to "...have the goodness to purchase two Girths, and a Sircingle and a Crupper." Should you not be familiar with these terms, they are articles of harness. In another letter John asks, "If you possibly can, send me 6 Ewes and 1 Ram. I have not tasted mutton for two years past and wish very much to raise a stock."[7]

So much for the home requirements and comforts of the pioneers. The *Nancy* also carried barrels of produce for the forts. As noted earlier, the Thames Valley was the breadbasket of the western outposts in those days, at least until laid waste by the Americans in 1813. After that, a great deal of the grain needed by the British was supplied by farmers on the American side, and smuggled across Lake Erie. The *Nancy* also carried the garrisons themselves, their cannon, powder and ball. She took part in the assault on Fort Stephenson on the Sandusky River in July, 1813. On August 1, she was cruising off Put-in-Bay. Mackintosh calls it "Pudding Bay" in his log, which can now be found in the library of McGill University in Montreal. On August 2, he sends ashore for some hay for the sheep. On the third, he is taking soundings at the entrance to the Sandusky.

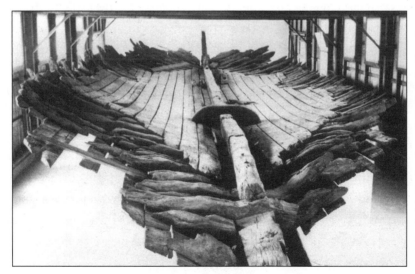

The remains of the keel and ribs of the Nancy *are on display at Wasaga Beach Provincial Park.* Courtesy of Nancy Island Historic Site, Wasaga Provincial Park.

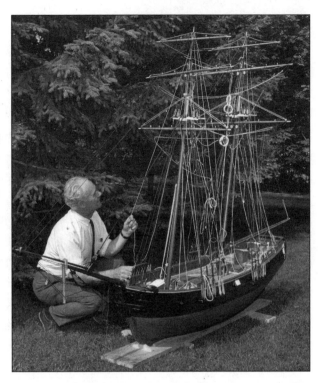

This model of the Nancy *was built in the 1920s by the gentleman in the picture, William Van Der Valk. It was donated to the Nancy Island Historic Site at Wasaga Beach and remains on display.* Courtesy of the Ontario Department of Tourism, now Ministry of Tourism.

The *Nancy's* activities were more or less mundane until that fateful day on which the American troops spotted her masts through the trees. She was destroyed, but not forgotten. In 1927, after lying underwater for 113 years, what remained was salvaged and raised. A small museum was built on the site to protect the artifacts from weather and vandals. In later years, other buildings were erected nearby, and a contemporary museum was opened in 1978. I can still remember seeing the charred remains of her hulk when my father took me there to see the wreckage in 1928. We rented a cottage at Wasaga Beach at that time, but shipwrecks did not make a meaningful impression upon the mind of a seven-year-old child, as I was then. They certainly do so today.

After the war was over, the North West Company claimed and received £500 pounds for two round trips of the *Nancy* from the Detroit River to Fort Erie. For her services in 1813-14, her owners were paid £1,243 .5s. 0 p. In addition, they received £1,200 as compensation for the loss of the vessel.

CHAPTER 14

The Story of *HMS St. Lawrence*

IMAGINE IF YOU WILL, a ship sweeping down Lake Ontario, her billowing sails reaching to the height of a twenty-storey building. Such a vessel was the *HMS St. Lawrence*, the largest and most powerful ship-of-the-line ever to operate on the Great Lakes. She was built at Point Frederick[1] (Kingston, Ontario) in no more than six months, and launched on September 10 in 1814. "Man has never built anything more beautiful than a full-rigged ship under a press of canvas."[2]

For a brief moment, she was the secret weapon of her time and place. The *St. Lawrence* never entered history for the battles she won. Her memory is preserved for the hostilities she prevented. She was even bigger than Lord Nelson's *Victory*.[3] When she was launched, all enemy ships returned to port and did not venture out again until after peace had been declared. Some writers credit her design to William Bell. Actually, British navy ships were of much the same design, differing only in size and few other details. A ship built in England and one built in Upper Canada would not differ greatly. However, the records show that Bell introduced many innovations in the construction. This was the result, in part, of a shortage of materials, for example, ship's knees. The draught from the records in the

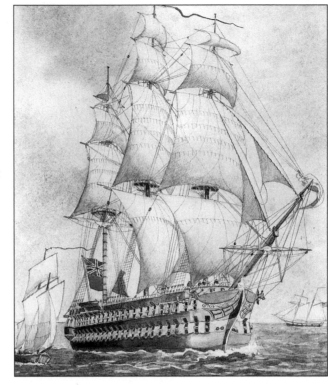

The HMS St. Lawrence *was the largest (in displacement) sailing vessel built on the Great Lakes. Constructed at the shipyard in Kingston and launched in September 1814, she commanded the lake.* C.H.J. Snider, *artist.* Courtesy of the TRL, JRR 1186.

National Maritime Museum was drawn and signed by Master Shipwright Thomas Strickland. It is dated at Kingston Naval Yard, May 1815, and is an "as built" draught.

We know little of designer William Bell's life, though what is known is all honourable and respectable. He was master shipwright at Amherstburg soon after the turn of the century and was responsible for building Robert Barclay's fleet. After the Battle of Lake Erie in 1813, the yards at Amherstburg were destroyed, and Bell moved to Kingston.

Sir James Yeo expressed his pleasure with his new flagship in a letter written to the Admiralty, "I believe the St. Lawrence has completely gained the Naval ascendancy on this Lake, and I am happy to say, she sails very superior to anything on it."[4] And David Wingfield wrote in his diary, "Our business from now to the setting in of winter was comprised in trying the sailing trim of the St. Lawrence, exercising the men at the guns, and supplying the different garrison with stores and provisions for their winter supply."[5]

Launched on September 10, the *St. Lawrence* did not put to sea until October 16, and made several trips up and down the lake, ferrying troops and supplies. But she never fired a gun in anger and her crew never saw the enemy from her decks. Actually, she came rather close to having a very short life indeed. On October 19, she had been in the water for little more than a month, when she was struck by lightning while on passage. The mainmast was damaged and several of the crew were killed. Fortunately, she was not out of service for more than a few days.

Once the Americans learned that a vessel of this exceptional size, capable of carrying 112 guns, was being built at Kingston, they started immediately to construct two ships of a size even bigger. They did make an attempt near Kingston harbour to destroy the *St. Lawrence* by blowing her up with a sort of torpedo, but the British chased the attackers away before they could accomplish anything. The weapon was really a floating mine, a powder keg with a harpoon for jabbing into the ship's side at or below the waterline. The British, in turn, started two more ships, the same size, to be named the *Canada* and the *Wolfe*, but they were never completed.

The two new American ships were to be the *New Orleans*, built at Sacket's and the *Chippewa* from nearby Storr's Harbor. They were to carry 120 guns each, but were never launched, due to the Rush-Bagot Agreement[6] initiated in 1816 by James Munroe and ratified by the United States and Britain in 1818. This agreement, defining

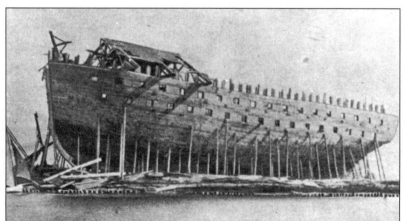

"Old Neverwet," the New Orleans *as she was in the 1870s. She was sold sometime around the mid-1880s and her timber used to make pencils.* Courtesy of the Archives of Ontario.

peace/disarmament terms, limited the naval force of the two countries to one ship each on lakes Ontario and Champlain, and two each on the Upper Lakes, thus ending the British/US naval race. All the British ships were laid up "in ordinary," a naval term meaning that all sails and rigging, guns, etc. were removed, except one. Sometimes the ship would be covered by a temporary roof to reduce weather damage. The Americans kept the *New Orleans* under commission until 1883, though they never finished her. She sat uncovered for a time, then a storehouse was built around her. Later she was sold, along with the storehouse to a manufacturer of pencils.

Thirty years after the Rush-Bagot agreement was signed, that is to say, in 1848, the hulk of the *St. Lawrence* was sold for £25. While some writers say this happened in 1832 and others suggest 1826, there seems to be some agreement that the hulk was sold in the mid-1800s. She is reported to have cost Britain £800,000. The ship was towed away from Navy Bay, the dockyard in Kingston, to a long limestone building west of Macdonald Park where they beached her. A gangway was built from the old harbour highway of King Street in Kingston and the noble *St. Lawrence* became a cordwood dock. Now, the steamers leaving Kingston for passage up or across the lake could load up with fuel. It is said that the hulk eventually slipped under the water where she had served as that fuel dock. Others say that she was towed away and sunk, perhaps in Deadman Bay or Navy Bay, where vandals could not humiliate her further. Where, in fact, does she lie now? If I did know I would not tell.

Some years ago, the Toronto printing house of Rous and Mann produced a promotion piece to aid in plans of persuading the Ontario government to raise the *St. Lawrence*, rebuild her and make a tourist attraction. The text, "The Silent St. Lawrence," and an excellent painting, were by C.H.J. Snider. It was long out of print when this story was being researched, but wonderfully helpful in providing much of the background information on the *St. Lawrence*.[7]

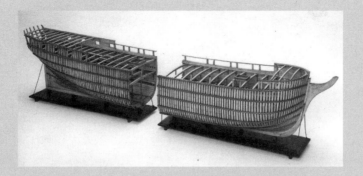

PART THREE

Shipbuilding in a Wilderness Setting

Bless and praise us famous men
Men of little showing
For their work continueth…
Great beyond their knowing. – Rudyard Kipling

Day by day the vessel grew,
With timbers fashioned strong and true,
Stemson and keelson and sternson knee,
Till, framed with perfect symmetry,
A skeleton ship rose up to view!
And around the bows and along the side
The heavy hammer and mallet plied,
Till after many a week, at length,
Wonderful for form and strength,
Sublime in its enormous bulk,
Loomed aloft the shadowy bulk!
From "The Building of a Ship," – Henry Wadsworth Longfellow

Model of a ship in frame. Courtesy of The Science Museum, London, England.

CHAPTER 15

Ship Construction in the Early 19th Century

"The history of wooden shipbuilding on the Great Lakes and the knowledge and skills of the men who were engaged in this early industry, is rapidly becoming lost sight of." Thus wrote Captain H.C. Inches in 1962, in introducing his book, *The Great Lakes Wooden Shipbuilding Era.* "Yet the history of Great Lakes shipping began with those vessels, which were built of wood, fashioned by men whose understanding of shipbuilding enabled them to construct, entirely by hand, vessels that were long-lived and seaworthy," he declared.[1] Captain Inches was 94 years of age when this statement was written. He had spent all his life in and among ships on the lakes, watching their construction in the yards as a master of Great Lakes bulk carriers, and considerable time as trustee and director of the Great Lakes Historical Society.

While there have been many books published in Europe on naval architecture and shipbuilding in the 18th and 19th centuries, books on ship construction in this period are very hard to find. It has not been possible to locate a comprehensive book on the methods and skills used in shipyards anywhere. It has been necessary to cull scraps of information from many books and articles, American,

British, French and Dutch, a bit here, a fragment there, and collect it together for this section.

Fortunately, North American shipyards and methods differed very little from contemporary yards in Europe. All the shipbuilding technology of the day originated in Europe. The French were considered masters of the art and the British and Dutch were not far behind. Many of the shipwrights in North American yards had emigrated from Europe. Even in early colonial days, yards had been established in the coastal communities and ships were built for the British navy in some of these yards well before the American Revolution.

In 1798, Josiah Fox, a 30-year-old shipbuilder emigrated from England, and the records show that he brought copies of the then-current reference texts for building ships with him. He had learned the trade, apprenticed to a master shipwright at the Plymouth Dockyard. Fox's training was superior to anything available in America at that time, and he had a hand in designing many frigates for the US Navy, which really was founded in 1794 when Congress passed an Act authorizing the construction of six frigates. Fox worked with Joshua Humphreys, one of the best known of the early American shipbuilders, and is credited with designing the *United States* and the *Constitution*. Similarly, several former officers of the Royal Navy in America changed their loyalty during the Revolution and served the War Office in Washington. As was noted earlier, Henry Eckford, a Scot, had learned the trade of shipwright in the yards at Quebec. And to him goes the credit for building the ships at Sacket's so quickly and efficiently.

There were naturally great similarities between the vessels built by American yards and British yards on the lakes. Most of the designs on the Canadian side originated with the Admiralty in London. Also, most of the skilled shipwrights and carpenters came out from England directly to the Kingston and Fort Malden shipyards. Furthermore, tools and equipment were essentially the same on both sides of the border. The comparative availability of personnel and equipment and, in particular, of armament, made up the principal differences.

Accessibility of supplies, including aged timber, was also a key difference between shipyards on the lakes and the Royal Navy dock-yards in England. This availability was most obvious in the early days of the war in the shortage of guns for the British vessels, but throughout the war, it became very apparent in the quality of timber. By the time that Britain had almost run out of oak trees, she was importing pine from Scandinavia. When the already high duties on Baltic timber were nearly doubled in 1811, thus pricing it out of the market, Britain turned to her North American colonies. Standing trees were in good supply in Upper Canada, though the infrastructure, such as roads for procuring timber, was much worse. The kits, however, for the *Canada* and the *Wolfe* were of fir, not oak.

While it was not possible to find any list of materials that were imported from England for the construction of the *St. Lawrence*. John Spurr, writing in *Queen's Archives*, gives the following list of material needed to build a 32-gun frigate, 126 feet by 35 feet:

600 tons of carefully selected and shaped timber.

40 tons of iron fittings, nuts and bolts.

12 tons of copper bolts

2,000 sheets of copper

18,000 treenails

1 ton of oakum for hull and deck seams

20 barrels of pitch

1 40 gallon barrel of tar

150 gallons of linseed oil

2.5 tons of paint [Note: presumed to be in liquid form]

15 tons of sails (standing rigging)

12 tons of sails (running rigging)

6 tons of wooden blocks

1 tons of spare yards and booms

40 tons of crafted wood (masts, yards and bowsprit)

35 tons of anchor cables

An unspecified tonnage of chains, hawsers and assorted ropes.[2]

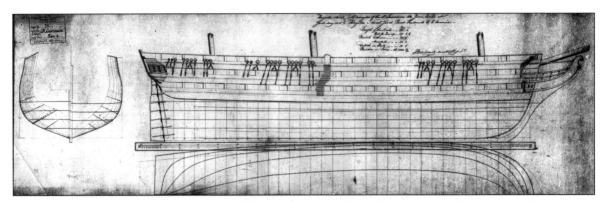

Draught of the HMS St. Lawrence *hull, as built by Thomas Strickland, Kingston, 1815.*
Courtesy of the National Maritime Museum, London, UK.

All but the timber products and the copper would have to be imported from England at very great difficulty of transport and expense. Bear in mind, this list applies to a vessel less than half the weight of the *St. Lawrence*, and to another venue, and the list does not include the guns, powder and shot. While British ships were coppered at this time, no copper was used in Upper Canada.

In England, during this time, a tree trunk was aged, subject to the exigencies of war, one year for each inch of its thickness. In the shipyards, in the early colonial period, a tree could be growing in the morning and be part of a ship's frame by the evening.

In Devonport, England, the keel for the 80-gun *HMS Foudroyant* was laid down in 1789, but she was not launched until 1798. It was desirable to let a vessel sit "in frame" for several years so that any warping or rot could be found and corrected before planking. It happened on occasion that the rot was so bad that the ship "in frame" had to be destroyed and was never finished. The *Foudroyant* had an unusually long life and was still afloat until destroyed by storm in 1897, ninety-nine years after her launching.

On the other extreme, the mighty *St. Lawrence* was started and launched in just one summer. She is being compared here with the *Foudroyant*, as there are many similarities in size and design. Also, there are photographs of the *Foudroyant*, which have been compared favourably with the only pictures of the *St. Lawrence* made during her lifetime. The draughts of both have been compared also, the principal difference being depth of hold, and therefore the draft of water needed to float them.

Foudroyant	*St. Lawrence*
Built Devonport, England, 1789-98	Built Kingston, Upper Canada, 1814 (6 months)
LOA 184'	LOA 191'
Beam 50' 6"	Beam 52' 5"
Displacement, 2,054 tons	Displacement 2,504 tons
Crew 650	Crew 640
Guns 80	Guns 112

I have a personal and direct interest in the *Foudroyant*. Following her destruction in a storm in 1897, some of her timbers were made into pieces of furniture and sold. In 1968, my wife Jean located a beautiful, heavy, oaken throne-chair, made from these timbers, and presented it to me as a loving gift. Furthermore, my next yacht, purchased in 1972, was christened, *Foudroyant*. She served me well until she was sold in Europe in 1999. We made many adventurous but safe passages together (mostly international), in both freshwater and saltwater, totalling over 25,000 miles.

The Shipyard

During time of war, the ability to defend the site from an enemy, either by land or sea, was essential. In addition, the site had to be near a body of water sufficiently deep to float the ship when completed. There were other requirements. The land must be firm and reasonably level, in close proximity to a source of good timber, and have access to other shipbuilding supplies. Suitable road or water transportation was a necessity, and finally, the transportation route had to be as safe as possible from attack and plundering by the enemy.

A supply of labourers was not so important. Men could be brought in if not available locally, as was done in all the shipyards of the lakes at this time. Hulks were sometimes converted into floating dormitories, as was done at Kingston. More often, bunkhouses were erected nearby, or the townspeople would accommodate the transients. The shipyards contributed greatly to the growth and economic development of the communities such as concern us here. In Kingston, many of the workers stayed after the war. At Erie and Sacket's Harbor, the majority returned to the seacoast.

Just a few buildings were required for the actual construction work. It was all completed out of doors, summer or winter. A room in a residence could be commandeered for administrative work. Sheds would be required for storage and for such work as sail-making, rigging and the like. A large covered area with a relatively smooth, flat floor was needed for lofting. And, of course, a forge was a necessity, although relatively little metal went into the construction of most of these ships. As time went on, additional buildings would be erected for such purposes as a joiner's shop where fittings were made, such as blocks, ship's wheels, furniture, figurehead, etc. A ropewalk would provide a real advantage.

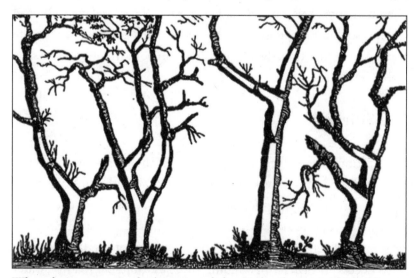

When choosing trees in the forest intended as timber for use in shipbuilding, one had to be able to visualize the naturally occurring "shapes" that could be obtained for the various structural components needed in the construction process. Sketch by James Somerville.

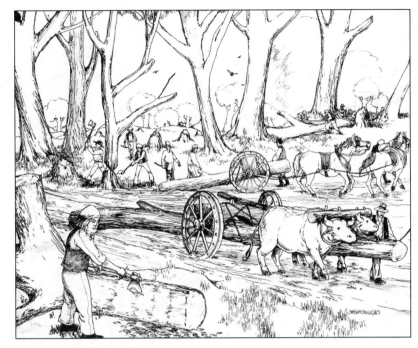

Cutting, trimming and hauling the timber to the shipyard. Sketch by James Somerville.

A sail loft needed a large, clean, floor area for laying out, measuring, cutting, sewing, roping and so on. There would be a cookhouse for the workers, stables for yard horses, blacksmith's shop and such services. The ships themselves were rarely built under roof.

The best timbermen would spend days wandering in the woods, selecting and marking the most suitable trees. They were selected for their natural shape where branches joined the trunk and would make natural knees, or for straight and curved planks or futtocks. The felled trees would be hauled to the yard by teams of oxen or horses, preferably in winter time. In fact, masts could only be hauled in winter. Due to their tremendous weight, no road of the day, only frozen earth, could bear their weight.

Some 3,000 loads of timber went into making the frames, knees, etc. of a first-rater, plus the planking, decking and spars. This would mean that upwards of 4,000 trees were felled to make one ship such as the *St. Lawrence* or the *New Orleans*. Oak was the preferable species for the frames, keel, knees and similar members, and, when available, was also used for planking. Ash was utilized for oars. White

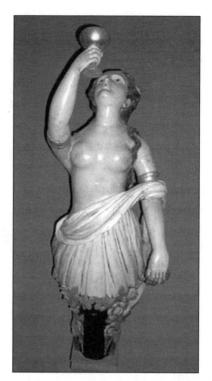

This figurehead is from a special collection housed at the Mystic Seaport Museum, Connecticut. While most of the depictions are of females, several show male figures of importance to the shipbuilder or owners. Figureheads have been used on the bows of sailing ships for centuries, as early as Egyptian and Grecian times. The first symbols used were the shapes of "eyes" to help wayward ships find their way. It is purported that the figures of women, especially nude women, were used to calm the angry seas. Courtesy of Paul Carroll.

pine was employed for decking. In North America, unseasoned wood was used most frequently, no other being available, and frequently various types of wood were applied side by side.

The ships of war were generally built "just good enough and no better than needed." Very little decoration or gilding was used, though the *Princess Charlotte* (a 44-gun frigate with a length of 121 feet on the gun deck, built in Kingston in 1814), was fitted with a figurehead. Commercial ships, built in peacetime, sometimes were much better constructed, and exhibited the vanity of the owners. The *Nancy*, and the *Hamilton* were so adorned with additional decoration, so as to suit their owners' fancies.

Pine for masts and other softwood could be transported in rafts. Oak could be hauled by ship but not floated to the yards due to its high density. It would sink if placed in water. In summer, trees would be hauled, slung under the axle of ox-carts with very large wheels, known as timber tugs. In winter, they would be carried on sleighs where the tree itself made up the frame of the sleigh. Many farmers increased their cash income by hauling timber all winter. They prayed for a hard winter and good sleighing.

In general there was no shortage of timber near all the yards at the beginning of the war, though as time went on, it was necessary to haul from further and further afield each winter. Along the seacoast, it was common to get curve-grained, oak compass timber from the live-oak groves in North Carolina and Georgia. These fine hardwoods were used in the Canadian Maritime Provinces, New England and New York consistently, but were not available for yards on the lakes. In late 1814, three sets of frames were sent out from England but were never used since the return to peace made them unnecessary.

The trees were felled using the woodsman's axe and cross-cut saw. Most early settlers were, of necessity, skilled in the use of these tools. The trees were selected for use as knees, frames or planks, and shaped using either the long ripsaw (whipsaw) or by the use of a broadaxe and an adze.

The Skills of the Ship Carpenters

Captain Inches, in writing about planking, states, "I have seen these large timbers joined with a lock joint so tight you could not slip a cigarette paper in at any place."[3] C.H.J. Snider, in one of his many articles, describes a man who placed his bare foot on a beam and with his

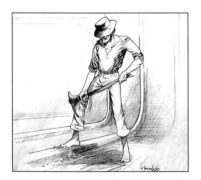 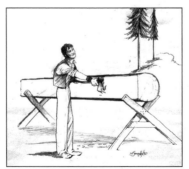 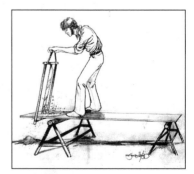

Both the felling of trees and the carpentry work required in the construction of ships called for exceptional skills in the use of tools. From left: working with an adze, working with a broadaxe and working with a ripsaw. All sketches by James Somerville.

adze shaved a piece of wood from under his sole as thin as a piece of tissue paper.

Captain Inches, while discussing mast-makers, declared, "I have seen these professionals stand on one of these logs, swing a ship-axe from the shoulder and split a chalk line mark."[4] F.W. Wallace, in his book *Ships of Wood and Men of Iron*, writes of Quebec ship carpenters who could split a playing card edgewise with the adze.

In continuing his description of shipbuilding, Captain Inches writes, "After the ship was planked, stem to stern and from keel to topside, the carpenters went to work and adzed down the entire planking. These men were artists with that tool and never made any deep gouges in the planks. Instead, they made the planks so smooth that the planing with a small plane was not a heavy job. They gave the ship a beautiful, smooth, finish outside."[5] The term for this skill with the adze was known as "dubbing." John E. Horsley, in *Tools of the Maritime Trades*, writes on the use of a ripsaw, a narrow blade type of pitsaw, "The frames were not just sawn out, but bevelled at the same time."[6] How closely could the bevels be cut? "To the thickness of a pencil line."

Steam-powered sawmills were beginning to appear in shipyards in England after 1793. Wind-driven sawmills had been in use a great many years but water-powered mills were rarely employed in shipyards in North America at this time. The machinery for these mechanical saws started with a crank on the end of the waterwheel shaft. This was connected to a pitman rod, then to a gate-saw in an upright frame that travelled vertically, in slides.

The records show that the sawmill closest to Erie was at Pittsburgh, some 130 miles away. However, there were none recorded at Sacket's. In Upper Canada there were several mills on streams flowing into the St. Lawrence River, at Cornwall, Prescott, etc., but too far away to be of much assistance. A gristmill and sawmill had been opened at Kingston Mills six miles up the Cataraqui River from Kingston in 1783, and another at Millhaven a few miles west of the town. These mills could not be expected to cope with the quantity of sawn timber needed at Kingston in 1812-15, so it must be assumed that a very large proportion of all sawing was done by hand. Circular saws and band saws had not been invented at the time of the War of 1812.

The Tools of the Shipwright

Woodworking tools changed very little down through the centuries preceding the advent of power. Rudyard Kipling[7] captured the scene in verse:

> I tell this tale which is strictly true,
> Just by way of convincing you
> How very little since things were made
> Things have altered in the shipwright's trade.

Many of the tools used 180 years ago in the shipyard are readily recognized in a rural, present-day carpenter's shop. Among them are the following:

Adze, lipped, plain and broad styles.
Axe, plain, broad and mast maker's, plus "lumber-man's."

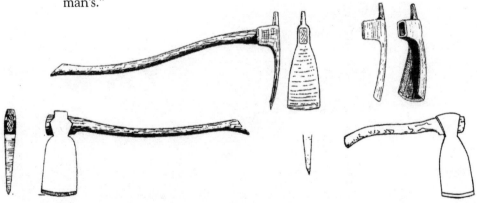

Top: The "plain" adze (top right) was usually used when cutting with the grain of the wood. The "lipped" adze (left) was used when cutting across the grain. Bottom: The broadaxe (right) and the mast maker's axe (left). Sketches by Heidi Hoffman.

Augur, not the present ratchet brace, but a simpler tool, similar to an oversize gimlet, and the long, shipwright's augur, or even the pod augur.

Various types of drill were in regular use: a) the common "carpenter's brace and bit"; b) a shell or "nose" augur, sometimes as much as three inches in diameter, also furnished with a shaft four feet long and with suitable handles for drilling through a keel and keelson; also known as a "pod augur"; c) a single twist augur, less common because of the danger of it getting stuck and breaking in the hole. Sketches by Heidi Hoffman.

a b c

Countersink, for enlarging holes that would later be plugged with wood.
Caulking irons, dumb and making.
Caulking mallet.

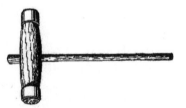
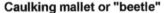

Caulking mallet or "beetle"

Caulking irons

Tools used in caulking. Sketches by Heidi Hoffman.

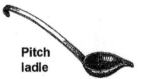

Pitch ladle

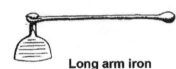

Long arm iron

Chisels, many shapes and sizes, up 2-1/2" face.
Clamps, or cramps, made of very heavy steel bar and able to open as much as 3-4 feet.
Draw knives, similar to today's tools, also referred to as draw-plane or spoke-shave
Gauges and dividers, for measuring and marking.

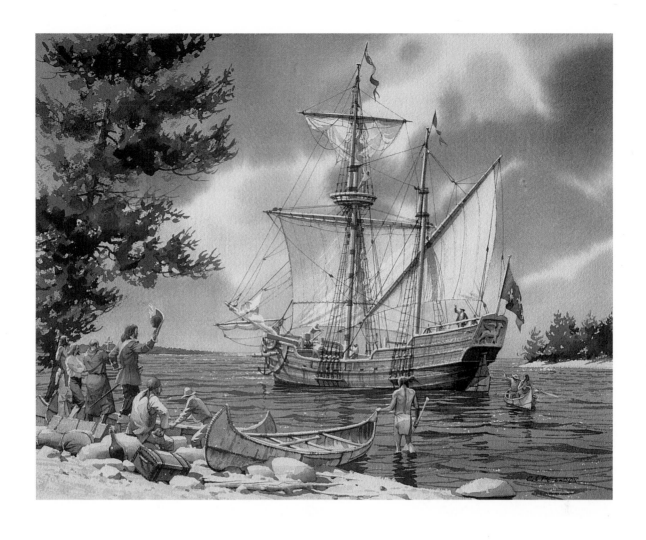

Charles L. Peterson
La Salle Waves "Bon Voyage," 1978
Watercolour
Courtesy of The Bamford Collection

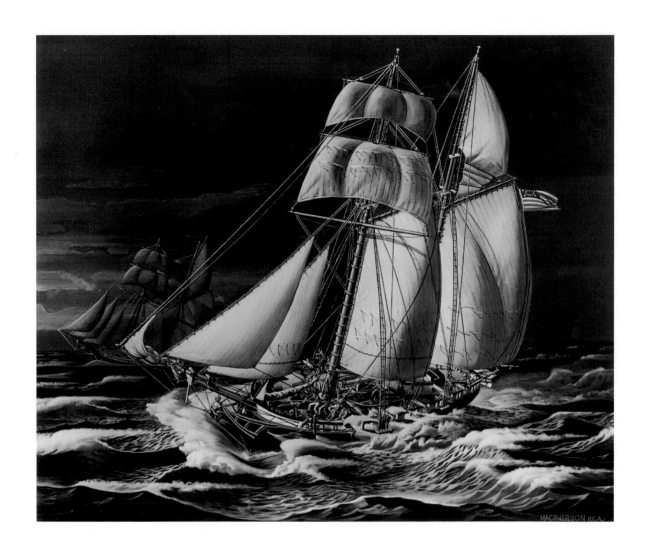

Duncan MacPherson
The Hamilton and the Scourge, 1982
Oil on canvas
Courtesy of Dorothy MacPherson

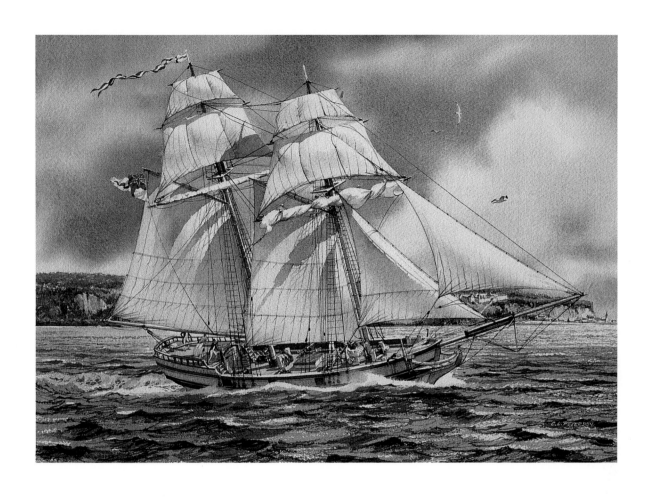

Charles L. Peterson
The Nancy Under Sail, 1980
Watercolour
Courtesy of The Bamford Collection

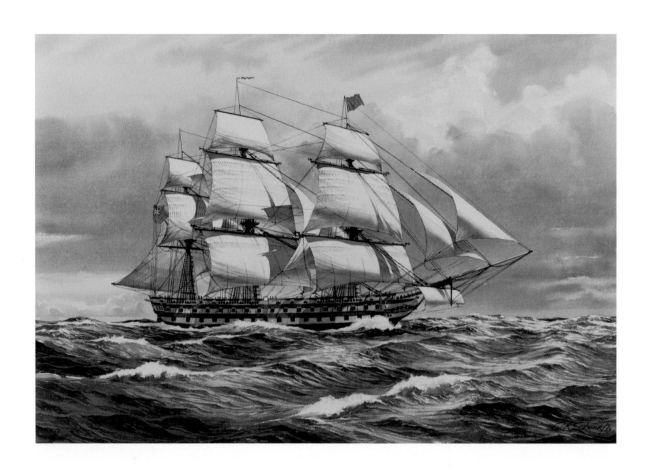

O.K. Schenk
The St. Lawrence, 1981
Watercolour
Courtesy of The Bamford Collection

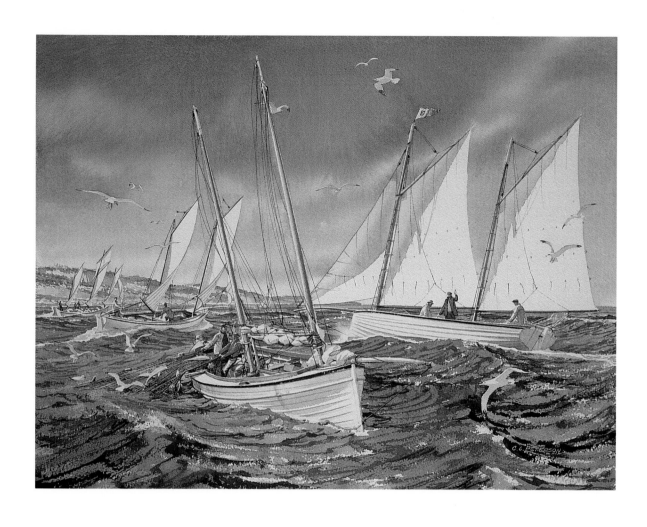

Charles L. Peterson
Fishing From Small Sailboats, 1982
Watercolour
Courtesy of The Bamford Collection

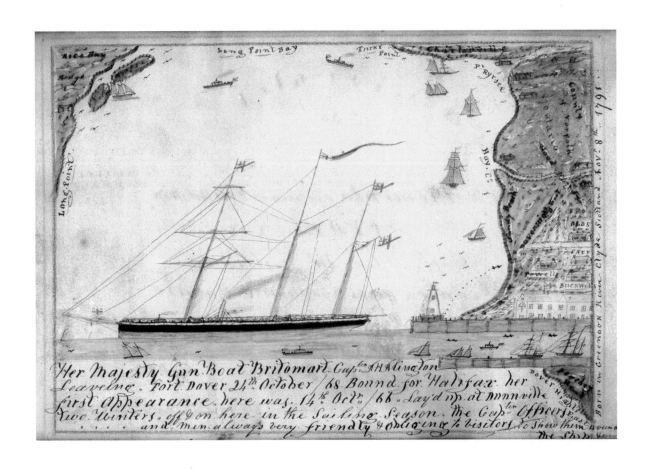

Captain Alexander McNeilledge
The HMS Britomart in Port Dover, 1868
Watercolour, ink and coloured pencil on paper
Courtesy of Mary Morrison

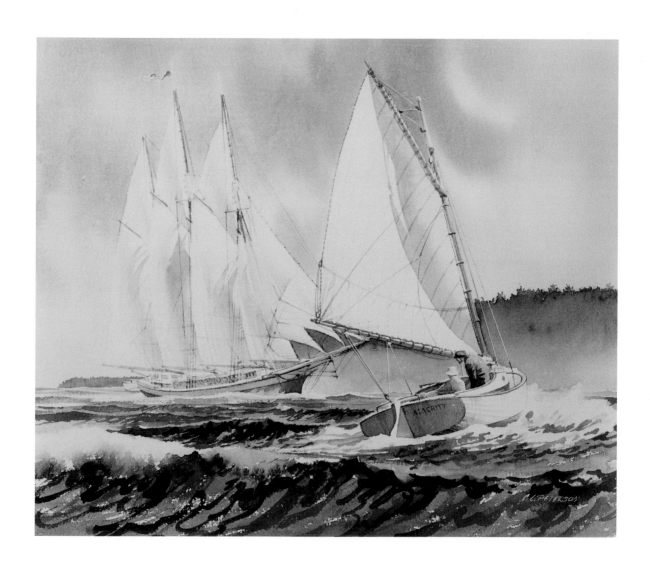

Charles L. Peterson
The Annie M. Peterson, 1972
Watercolour
Courtesy of The Bamford Collection

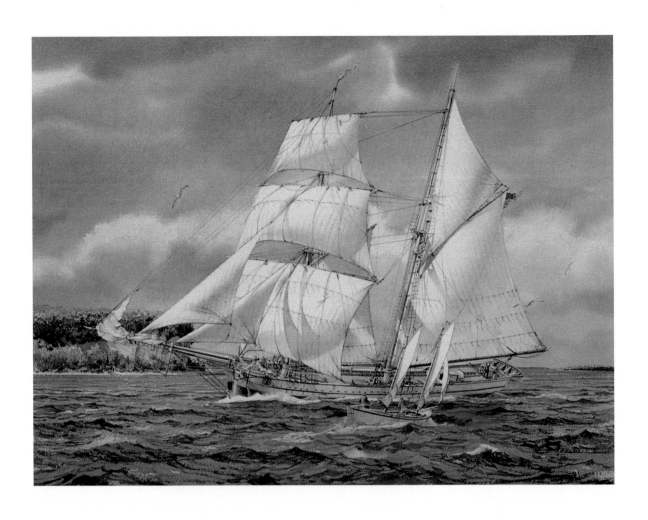

Charles L. Peterson
The Alvin Clark, 1983
Watercolour
Courtesy of Charles L. Peterson

Gin pole, a long wooden pole with a pointed tip, used primarily to assist in holding timbers and frames up while they are being fastened in place.

Hammers, ball pien, claw and mallets.

Moot, a form of plane for making treenails.

Oilstone (an abrasive stone used for sharpening tools),

Peavey, a heavy wooden lever with a pointed steel tip and a hinged hook near the end, used for moving logs and baulks, e.g. on the sawpit.

Planes, hollowing curved (for mast making), common smoothing plane, Jack planes, large (28" long), and small.

Plumb bob and line.

Saws, cross cut, compass, hack, rip (whip).

Spirit level, ship carpenter's.

Squares, long armed, large steel.

Nearly all planking was sawn by hand and all heavy material was shaped and fitted by use of adze, broadaxe and plane. Sawing planks was a laborious process. A pit was dug and a staging set up across it. The log was levered out on the staging and sawn by the use of a long, two-man handsaw, similar to the timberman's crosscut saw. One man stood on the staging, astraddle the log and facing opposite to the direction of the saw cut. He was responsible for the accuracy of the cut. The man in the pit faced the direction of the saw cut to try to reduce the amount of sawdust falling on his head, and by alternately pulling on the saw, the men could rip a log into a plank. The work was slow and required so much skill that the role of sawyer became a recognized trade. A gang usually consisted of the top sawyer and his helper, the pit sawyer, or pitman, with a third man whose job it was to shift the log at intervals using a peavey, (a long pole ending in a metal spike and hinged hook) so the saw could clear the staging, or to reposition the log to start a new cut.

Sawing planks with a pit saw. Note the positions of the two men. Sketch by James Somerville.

This was also the usual method of sawing compass timber or cutting large timbers and planks, also called fletches. Cutting wide planks into narrower pieces, or further shaping for compass timbers would be done by a rib saw, also called a turning saw or a futtock saw. Much of the shaping of timbers, both plank and heavy, structural pieces, futtocks, knees, and so on, was done by the broadaxe or the adze. The skill of the men in this work has been described earlier

One striking difference between the information available to the builder then and now is found in use of plans. In the early days, the builder was expected to work from one plan or draught, together with the instructions or specifications, based on standard practice. Nowadays, the piles of drawings needed to build a battleship would almost sink any of Yeo's smaller warships.

Spar or rigging drawings were not furnished, nor were sail plans. They were all based on the "Establishment," an all-encompassing word originating in the Royal Navy much earlier, and meaning, in this context, "standard practice." Many of the ships built in Upper Canada for the war were constructed to Admiralty draughts. The rules were rigid, hard and fast, covering everything connected with the building and maintenance of ships that were rated according to the number of guns that they were intended to carry. A first-rate ship carried 100 guns, a second-rate 90, a third-rate 60 to 80, and so on.

From these draughts, full-size drawings of the ship's frames would be made on the loft floor, a process referred to as lofting. Moulds or patterns in thin planking were then made of each frame and all the necessary markings, such as the deck levels, were transferred to the moulds. Each frame would be made up of several pieces, known as futtocks. Thus, the moulds must also be made up of as many pieces. The member that ended up being laid across the keel was known as the floor.

Accuracy was a matter of training and skill, and actually much of this construction was apt to be rather crude with fairing done by eye. Hence, there was considerable variation in ships built from the same draughts.

All the records uncovered in researching this material show that the naval vessels of the time were launched stern first, though

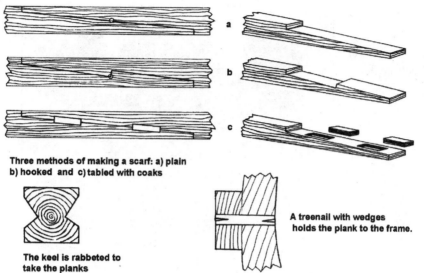

Three methods of making a scarf: a) plain
b) hooked and c) tabled with coaks

The keel is rabbeted to
take the planks

A treenail with wedges
holds the plank to the frame.

Scarfs, coaks, a rabbeted keel and a treenail. Sketches by Heidi Hoffman.

some commercial ships were launched broadside. The building slip, or slipway, had to be very strongly built to support a weight of the finished hull – perhaps 1,000 tons – for the duration of the construction, then to withstand the strains of launching the vessel. The slipway was built, extending at right angles to the water's edge, for a length to accommodate the keel and a bit more, and it would be sloped between 3/8" and 1" per foot of length. It may have been made by laying huge timbers, parallel to the water's edge, imbedded in the earth, each some 30 to 40 feet in length and three to six feet apart. On that bed would be placed cribs of squared timbers, to a height of five feet or more, so that the men could work under the keel. At the top of each crib, a cap of straight-grained oak was secured with the grain running parallel to the long axis of the slipway. Above these hefty cribs, the keel would be laid and the ship would be built. As the frames were raised, and as the hull was planked, props or shores were fitted beneath to spread the weight and take some of it off the cribbing.

The keel was fashioned of white oak. Several pieces were joined together by means of a joint called a scarf (also spelled scarph) ten to twenty feet in length. The scarfs were on the horizontal plane and were usually tabled or coaked. Coaks were generally square or rectangular inserts and did not replace the treenails. The keel might consist

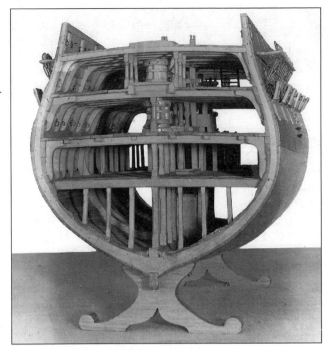

A model from an earlier era of sailing vessel. Note how the outside planks increase in thickness at the widest point. These are the "wales." Note how the inside planks, known as the ceiling, change thickness where each deck joins the walls. Note the wooden knees. There are many construction details here. Courtesy of The Science Museum, 5028 (London, UK).

of seven or more pieces, each about 30 feet in length, or longer, to allow for the scarfs. To prevent leaks along the seam of a scarf, a hole was drilled across the seam and a softwood dowel was driven in. These dowels were called stopwaters. The keel would be "sided" 21 inches in the middle, tapered to about 19 inches at the stem and 16 inches at the stern, and would be 21 inches thick. These dimensions are for a ship the size of the *St. Lawrence* or the *New Orleans*.

In the larger vessels, timbers were not available of sufficient thickness for the depth of keel needed. The keel was then built up of two or more layers as in today's laminated construction. Scarf joints were always staggered for strength. Everywhere two timbers were fayed (or fitted) together, so that the flat surfaces were completely in contact, for example, the laminating of the keel or of futtocks in a rib. Where scarfing of two or more of these was necessary, the scarfs must be as far removed from one another as possible. This distance was known as the "shift" and was essential, for had the joints coincided or been laid adjacent to one another, the structure would have been weakened. The "Establishment" laid down rules for this spacing requirement.

The stern assembly has many pieces. The planking comes right to the stern post. Sketch by Heidi Hoffman.

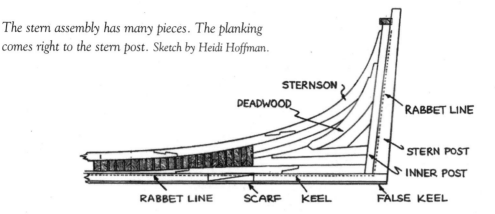

A false keel was usually attached later, beneath the keel, after the frames and the keelson were in place. It was deliberately made frangible, or capable of being broken, so that should the ship take the ground, the false keel might be ripped off but would prevent damage to the main keel itself. The keel would be temporarily secured to the underlying blocks with spikes or treenails on each side so that it could not shift sideways during construction.

Treenails, pronounced "trunnels," were made of well-seasoned oak or locust, sometimes circular, sometimes 16-sided. They varied in size from 1" to 1 3/4" in diameter and were hammered into holes slightly smaller in diameter so that, when they got wet and swelled, they formed a very strong fastening, generally leak-free. Wedges were driven in to the treenails at both ends, which helped make a very secure fastening.

The stern post was the next piece to be cut and put in position. It would be made up of pieces about 30 feet long and 26 inches square at the top, tapering to the bottom to a width of the keel but widened fore and aft to about 36 inches. It was mortised into the keel and set up vertically, when viewed from fore and aft, but raked aft, when viewed from the side. Solid filler pieces of oak, called deadwood, were laid on the keel aft of where the hull narrows, each piece treenailed to the next, and the lot, to the stern post. There might be 10 or 12 pieces of deadwood fitted into the stern. In similar fashion, the stem would be added next and it too would be made of several pieces of

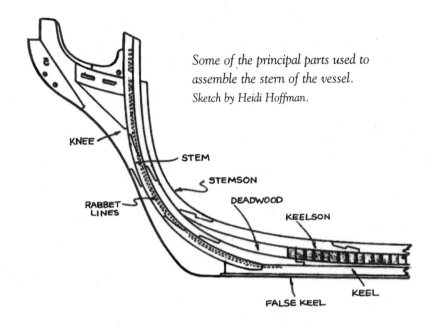

Some of the principal parts used to assemble the stern of the vessel.
Sketch by Heidi Hoffman.

KNEE

STEM

STEMSON

DEADWOOD

KEELSON

RABBET LINES

KEEL

FALSE KEEL

oak, scarfed together and treenailed, with fewer pieces of deadwood. The frames at the ends would later be set into notches or boxes cut into the deadwood.

The bows of vessels of this era would appear to us today to be extremely blunt in shape, almost "apple-cheeked." In profile they appeared much sharper but this was due to fashion pieces attached forward of the stem comprising the gripe and "beak head." It was not until the advent of the clipper ships that ships started to have a sharp entry. However, even at this time, some of the American ships were showing a much sharper entry than those of the British fleet.

Before any of the pieces of keel, stem or stern post were fastened together, they were rabbeted (or notched) as necessary. This means that the wood was cut out forming an angular groove to take the outside planking, the lowest or garboard strake (A strake is a row of planks from stem to stern; the garboard strake is the plank nearest to the keel.) This extensive, tedious and, of necessity, precise work was done by broadaxe and adze, finished off with chisel and mallet.

The stern post and stem were obviously very heavy timbers. They had to be hoisted into place using crude cranes consisting of A-frames, called "sheer legs" in those days, with a sturdy block and tackle. As soon as erected, the parts would be carefully lined up, plumbed and then shored so rigidly that they could not possibly shift from their correct position as the work progressed.

The ship's frames, of white oak, were made up of overlapping pieces, called "futtocks" fastened together, and cut from grown shapes or compass timber. Fourteen or more pieces might be used in a single frame assembly, each piece scarfed to the next above and below, or joined by chocks. Scarfs, of course, had shift, and all were treenailed. A midship frame was a gigantic U-shaped configuration, the bottom of which, rather flat, crosses over the keel. The laminated beam would be some eight inches thick and up to 24 inches in width, fore and aft, according to Establishment rules. Not all frames were laminated. Many were single frames, especially in way of the gun ports.

The spaces between the frames were frequently about half the width of a frame timber. The word "frame" and the word "rib" seem to have been interchangeable. In large vessels it appears that the floor pieces were first installed and lined up accurately. The half-frames were assembled on a platform or on level ground and reinforced with battens and with planks nailed over the chocks, to be removed later. Both port and starboard frames would be raised at the same time,

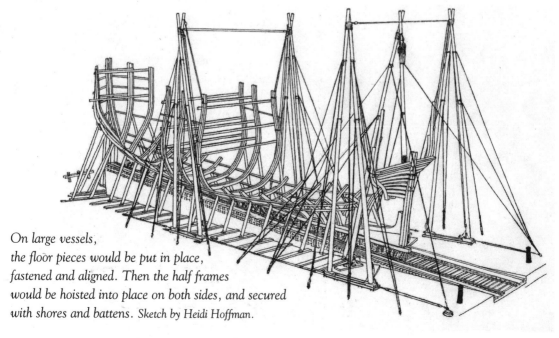

On large vessels, the floor pieces would be put in place, fastened and aligned. Then the half frames would be hoisted into place on both sides, and secured with shores and battens. Sketch by Heidi Hoffman.

using the block and tackle, sheer legs and shores, and possibly assisted by windlasses and even animals to take the load.

On smaller vessels, a different technique was used. A temporary assembly platform, or framing stage, was built up across the keel. On this stage, the frame would be assembled under the supervision of the master shipwright. Since the frames were 15 to 30 feet across and up to 30 feet high, the platform must be at least this size. It would be moved along the length of the ship as the work progressed. Framing commenced near amidships where a few frames were essentially identical, but as the work progressed forward or aft, every frame became different. As the ends were approached, the curve of the shape became so extreme that it was necessary to set the frame at an angle so as to present a flat surface to the planking. This work required complex cutting where these frames joined the keel fore and aft. These were known as cant frames. Exceptional skill was required in this work.

After assembly on the platform, the frame was reinforced with cross spalls near the top, and the frame and keel were notched to

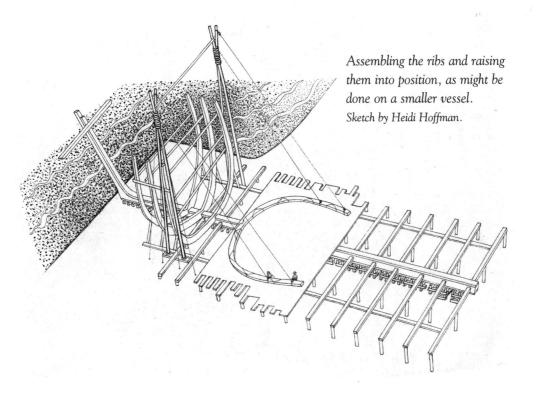

Assembling the ribs and raising them into position, as might be done on a smaller vessel.
Sketch by Heidi Hoffman.

accept one another. The frame was then raised into place and positioned across the keel.

Imagine what the weight of one of these frames must have been! Surely it would be upwards of several thousand pounds. Cranes were exceedingly simple A-frames, or jib-boom varieties, and, as noted, the heavy lifting was done by block and tackle. Sometimes, just workers, or possibly horsepower or oxen, contributed to sharing the load. The carpenters, with gin poles, would help line a frame up, and fit it into place. The frame, once in place, and made perpendicular to the keel, that is to say, off the vertical by the same angle that the keel made to the horizontal, is secured temporarily with spalls and ribbands, with battens sprung and fastened to a number of frames. "Spalls," "battens" and "ribbands" are names for pieces of timber used as a temporary support for parts such as frames while being erected until they are reinforced by planks.

As framing neared completion, the spaces between the cant frames at bow and stern would be filled in solidly, or very nearly so, with pieces of oak. There would be ten or so cant frames at each end of the ship. Once the frames were all in place and thoroughly faired by eye, the keelson was installed.

The "keelson" is a strengthening timber laid on top of the frames inside the vessel and through-bolted to the keel. Like the keel, it would consist of many scarfed timbers, possibly two or more layers thick, and with sister keelsons at each side. In a

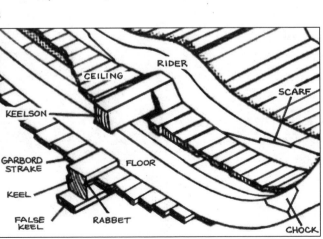

KNEE
GUNPORT
CEILING
CHOCK
RIDER
FUTTOCK
PLANKING
FLOOR
KEELSON
KEEL

RIDER
CEILING
SCARF
KEELSON
GARBORD STRAKE
FLOOR
KEEL
FALSE KEEL
RABBET
CHOCK

The backbone of the vessel was the keel, along with the keelson. Shown here is a typical assembly of keel, planking, floor, keelson, rider and ceiling. Sketch by Heidi Hoffman.

large ship such as the *St. Lawrence*, the keelson was a massive timber indeed. We have no record of the size of the keelson in the *St. Lawrence*, but in clipper ships, half the size of her displacement, it sometimes consisted of eight baulks, each 15 inches square.

This through-bolting was done with iron rods, shipped from England, driven in to a slightly undersized hole and headed over, at each end, onto a flat steel burr or washer. Drilling for these bolts, through four to six feet of wet oak, using primitive tools, must have been back-breaking work. It required a frequent change of labourer as the drilling progressed, hour after hour, day after day.

Now planking could commence. It started amidships, from the keel upwards and from the gunnels downwards simultaneously. The last planks to be put in, near the turn of the bilge were called the "shutter planks." Where plank ends met or butted, there had to be a frame. There must be at least three planks between butts on the same frame and no butts closer together than five feet from each other on consecutive planks. The planks had to be hung in close contact at the inside edge and were bevelled at the outside. The required bevel was approximately 1/16" to the inch of seam depth in order to take the caulking.

Before planking, the frames must be dubbed with an adze, that is to say, their outside surface faired so that the plank fitted tight against the frame. The planks were then lifted into place and sprung, edge set and twisted against the frames and tightly clamped against the edges of planks already in place. Chains, jacks, shores, clamps, the dangerous albeit ubiquitous Spanish windlass and wedges were used for this taxing work. The planks at bow and stern would have to be steamed because of the great curvature.

Dubbing ribs so the planks may be set tight against them. Drilling planks and driving in the treenails. Thousands of treenails would be used on one of these large vessels. Sketch by Heidi Hoffman.

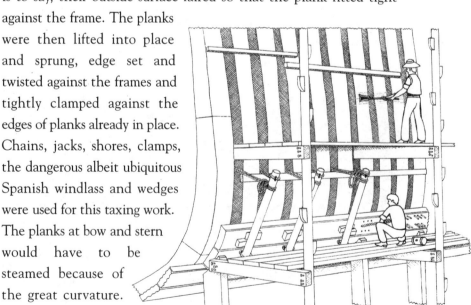

Before the advent of steam boilers and steam boxes, the planks would be thoroughly soaked and placed over a fire. Later, steam boxes, as long as sixty feet in length by three feet square, placed on both sides of the ship, and even inside, were commonly used. At the cry of "Hot plank!" the workers would drop their tools, and rush to carry the plank from the fire or steam box, up the ramp and on to the catwalk to where it was to be placed. They would protect themselves from being burned with old clothes, sacks, shavings or whatever was available.

Planks varied in thickness from sheer to keel, but would run to some four to eight inches thick and be of the same width. Imagine the weight of such a plank! Consider the problems of handling such a plank, hot from the fire, up the ramp, moving it along shaky catwalks and clamping it into position before it cooled. The uppermost plank would be many feet above the ground. Thicker planks, called gunwales or wales, were placed near the point of maximum beam, from stem to stern.

The plank, when finally in position, would be drilled and treenails were driven in, fastening it to the frames. Typically, six to eight treenails, 1 3/4" in diameter, or larger, would hold each plank at each frame. After cutting off any excess of the treenail, its end would be split and a wedge driven in to prevent the planks from pulling loose. Tens of thousands of such treenails would be pegged into place in a large vessel. The tool used was a wooden mallet, somewhat like a croquet mallet, though with a much shorter handle. The ceiling, heavy planking laid on the inside face of the frames, further strengthened the ship. Although not as thick as the outer planking, in total, the walls of the ship could be up to two feet thick.

Under each deck, on the inside of the hull are the fore and aft clamps, heavier timbers than the ceiling, on which rest the deck beams. The deck beams, tying the ship together athwartships, were also exceedingly heavy members, and spaced quite close together. Under each is a hanging knee in a vertical plane and alongside each is a lodging knee in the horizontal plane. The knees are all grown shapes made from oak compass timber.

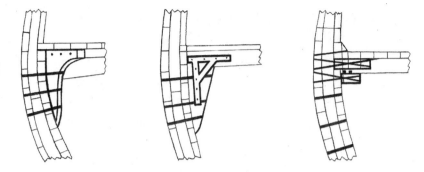

Three different types of metal knees. Grown knees (obtained from trees) became more difficult to obtain in English yards and substitutes such as these were in use by around 1800. Sketch by Heidi Hoffman.

Ordinarily in the early 1800s, a ship like the *St. Lawrence* would have some 400 knees. Archaeological divers have determined, however, that relatively few knees were used, and that William Bell, master shipwright at Kingston during the building of the *St. Lawrence,* had incorporated other innovations as well. British yards were acknowledging the shortage of naturally grown knees, and of oak suitable for shipbuilding generally. Bell employed a system that used far fewer wooden knees, for there were not sufficient of them at his site. He devised several forms of steel angles, which were being used in England about this time when grown knees, as noted, were in short supply. Furthermore, while earlier ships of war had the ribs spaced less than one-to-one with the air between them, as depicted in the model shown on page 129, it seems that ribs of most of the Great Lakes' vessels were spaced much further apart. Deck planking would probably be of pine, four to six inches thick, bevelled for caulking and fastened to the beams by means of treenails. In later ships, spikes or bolts, countersunk and plugged with wooden plugs would have been employed for fastening the deck planks in place.

Caulking the miles of seams was a tremendous job in itself. The caulkers used oakum and pitch. Oakum consists of hemp fibres made by unravelling old rope. Pitch was made from the sap of coniferous trees, probably imported from Scandinavia, to England, then to Canada. Sometimes caulking was hammered into place as many as three times over. Skilled caulkers did little else in the shipyard. Each had his own selection of irons, some curved, some straight, some broad, some narrow. In some of the smaller yards around the lakes, the skilled caulkers were in great demand, being contracted from place to place for larger shipbuilding jobs.

The blow of the caulking mallet produced a distinct musical note for the caulker would cut slots in the mallet, each differently, to create the note he wanted. The musical play of the caulkers' mallets was one of the most characteristic sounds of the shipyard. Author Stanley T. Spicer wrote in his book, *Masters of Sail*, "The never-to-be-forgotten sounds of those lovely summer mornings still ring in my ears. The sharp 'click' of the fastener's maul as the bolts were secured, the loud and merry ring of the caulker's mallet, the 'thub, thub' of the dubber's adze, the muffled blows on treenails, the swishing of broad axes, the whining saws, the hissing, sputtering steam-box when the steamed planks were withdrawn, combined in a jubilation of shipyard noises."[8] Others add to this the "geeing and hawing" of the drivers as they brought the loads of timber in by horse or ox-cart. It was a medley of sounds none of us will ever hear again.

As mentioned, sheathing the bottom with copper was not done on vessels for the Great Lakes, though the bottom would likely have been payed (painted on) with tar whenever it was available.

Launching was a day of celebration. A holiday would be declared and all the school children and townspeople would attend. Flags, bunting and speeches would be the order of the day, and the celebration would last well into the night. A military band might be provided to entertain the watchers while the vessel was being prepared for launching. A great deal of care was required for the successful launching of a 200-foot, 2,000-ton hull, or even a smaller one for that matter. In the interests of safety, celebration and libations among the workers were delayed as much as possible until after the event.

For several days, preparations were under way. First, the launching ways were built up under the ship, on heavy piles driven into the ground, or large piles of heavy timbers. The ways would be 10 to 15 feet on each side of the keel and very heavily constructed and shored. On top of these, other timbers were placed. Then a cradle was built, some 60 to 70 feet long, using these long timbers and cross braces. They were built up to the bottom of the vessel and kept from spreading by

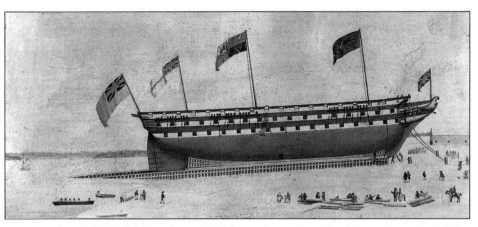

Launching day, artist not identified. Courtesy of the Royal Ontario Museum, 74 Can 258, 967-106-1.

passing and tightening cables or ropes under the ship. Next, the entire cradle was raised by driving wedges between it and the ways, thus taking the weight off the keel blocks and transferring the weight of the ship to the ways. The top of the ways and the bottom of the cradle were greased generously with tallow. Now time was short, for the vessel must be launched before the tallow was forced out by the ponderous weight of the ship resting upon it.

Just prior to launching, carpenters ventured beneath the ship. Using iron wedges and working from stern to bow, they gingerly split out the blocks on which the keel rested. As the last of the keel blocks was knocked out, the vessel would give a shudder, the carpenters would scramble to safety and the vessel would begin to move. Slowly at first, then faster as she gathered momentum, the vessel slewed down the ways and splashed into the water amid the cheers of the crowd and with the ways smoking from the friction.

> Then the Master with a gesture of command,
> Waved his hand, And at the word,
> Loud and sudden there was heard,
> All around them and below,
> The sound of hammers, blow on blow,
> Knocking away the shores and spurs,

And see! She stirs!
She starts – she moves – she seems to feel
The thrill of life along her keel,
And, spurning with her foot the ground,
With one exulting, joyous bound,
She leaps into the ocean's arms!
And lo! From the assembled crowd
There rose a shout, prolonged and loud,
That to the ocean seemed to say,
Take her, O bridegroom, old and gray,
Take her to thy protecting arms,
With all her youth and all her charms![9]

The ship would be immediately towed to the fitting-out berth. Joiners worked on the cabins aft and fitted partitions, furniture and such, although this generally would be very limited in a ship-of-the-line, especially on one for the Great Lakes. While the hull was being built, the spars would be made and assembled in readiness, in another corner of the yard. Spar making was a separate trade, but the skills were much the same. The tools used were the broadaxe, adze, drawknives and the spar plane.

There was no shortage of good pine in the vicinity, though it would have to be collected during the winter as the frozen ground would support the much heavier load. The best would have been selected and felled, straight and free from defects, then hauled in on sleighs by teams of oxen. It would be hewed out, flat on one side, with broadaxe and adze, then marked out with the proper taper. Following this procedure, it would be rolled and marked again, then cut to produce a four-sided, properly tapered timber. Now, using a spar-maker's gauge, it would be marked for cutting to eight sides. Then the process was repeated giving it sixteen sides, then planed to round. The finished spar would be painted, varnished or oiled.

The mainmast, for the ship under discussion, would be 123 feet from step to cap, foremast 8/9 of this, and mizzen 6/7. All lengths of masts and yards were derived from the Establishment formulae, from the length of the mainmast, as were the dimensions of the mainmast itself, to the top masts and topgallant masts. The diameter of the mainmast at the partners was about 37 inches and of the main yards at the slings about 24 inches. They were very substantial timbers indeed!

Stepping all the masts (putting them in their proper places in the ship) was straightforward, albeit dangerous, work for a ship's rigger of the day, using sheer legs on deck, or ashore with a multitude of block and tackle. Riggers made up the heavy standing rigging that held up the spars. There is no record of a ropewalk at Kingston, so presumably the rigging came from England, or the American seacoast. All standing rigging of the period was hemp, parcelled, served, and well-tarred.

Running rigging of hemp or manila (a strong fibre), for hoisting and trimming the sails, was rove through the blocks, and the sails bent on (attached to the masts and yards). Sails also had to be imported from England to Kingston, as well as brought into the American yards on the lakes. Sailcloth was already being manufactured on the seacoast in Boston. (The biggest source of sailcloth in the USA today is still Boston.) Sacket's Harbor had a sail loft, but the date it was first used has not been determined.

Ballast and stores would be loaded and stored below. All the armaments would be hoisted aboard and properly assembled on the carriages and their tackle rigged. When not "cleared for action," the guns were secured hard against the ship's walls or bulwarks so that they could not move around in a seaway. A gun broken loose and dashing about uncontrolled on a wild trip across the deck could leave a trail of death and destruction before crashing through the bulwarks into the lake. Here is born the expression, "like a loose cannon."

When one considers, that in the race for superiority on the lake, the *St. Lawrence* was built from standing timber to her launching in four to six months, and was ready for action in one more month, the magnitude of the project is amazing.

Although this chapter primarily describes the construction of a ship such as the *St. Lawrence* at Kingston in 1814, an even greater rate of shipbuilding took place at Sacket's Harbor in the winter of

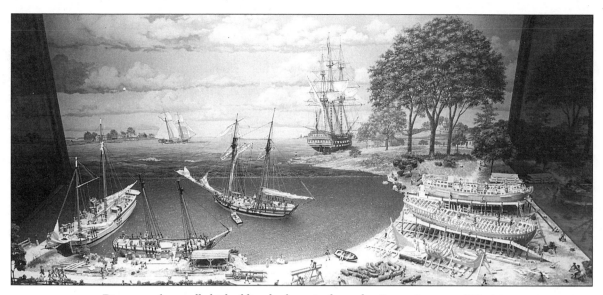

Diorama of a small shipbuilding harbour in the early 1800s. Courtesy of The Mariner's Museum, Newport News, Virginia.

1814-15. Chauncey certainly knew of the *St. Lawrence* long before she was launched, but it was not until November 1814, that he recommended the construction of three even larger first-class ships-of-the-line, a British naval term referring to a three-decked, fully armed first-rate ship. During the winter, they laid down the keels for two such ships, intended to carry up to 120 guns each, the *New Orleans* and the *Chippewa*. As noted, neither of these was ever launched. Similarly, at Kingston two more ships-of-the-line were started, the *Wolfe* and the *Canada*, both intended to carry 120 guns. They, too, were never launched.

On March 1, 1815, word reached Kingston that the treaty of peace had been ratified. Yeo promptly resigned his commission and headed home to England, travelling through the United States, stopping off at Sacket's Harbor on the way. He was impressed at the progress that had been made. "They more than half finished two ships of 120 guns each," he wrote.[10]

Lieutenant David Wingfield RN visited Sacket's Harbor in mid-June 1815, as a tourist. In fact, he sailed across from Kingston in a small pleasure boat. He had an opportunity to examine the two large ships, which had been partially built. This is the first known account of a pleasure cruise across Lake Ontario. He wrote, "The two ships on the stocks which, had they been launched, would have been larger, and carried more guns than any ship in the British navy; the largest was pierced for 150 guns, and the other would have been scarce ten guns short of that. The largest of the two on the stocks at Kingston would have mounted 136 and her consort 130 guns, thus, had the war continued, the mill pond Lake Ontario, compared with the ocean, would have had the largest ships in the world, or perhaps the largest ever built, upon the bosom of its waters… the largest American ship …her proportions were beautiful – the Americans at this time certainly beat all our ships in symmetry."[11]

Colonel J. Bouchette of the British Army also visited Sacket's Harbor, just a few months earlier, and reported that the American ships were finished with "no other polish than what is given them by the axe and the adze and were rushed into the water in about a month from the time the trees were standing in the forest." The ships built at Kingston were reported to be finished up to the standards of British ocean vessels, but also were built of green timber.

The shipyard at Sacket's Harbor in the winter of 1814-15 had been much more productive than that at Kingston. The credit for this goes to Henry Eckford and the Browns. However, this is not to say that Captain Conor, John Dennis, William Bell and Thomas Strickland, and the others at Kingston, were any less competent. In fact, the British accomplishment at Kingston was superior when one considers that everything that went into the ships, unless made of wood, had to be brought over from England.

With much fairness, Theodore Roosevelt wrote in *The Naval War of 1812*, summing up the year 1814 on Lake Ontario, "The success of the season was with the British, as they held command over the lake for more than four months, during which time they could co-operate with their army while the Americans held it for barely two months and a half."[12] He had pointed out in his book how much the US Army had failed to cooperate with the Navy, or was it the other way around?

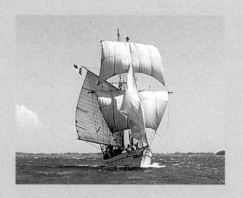

PART FOUR

Commercial Sail on the Lakes
Until the Early 1900s

*"I remember…the beauty and mystery of the ships
And the magic of the sea."* – Henry Wadsworth Longfellow

*"The fore-and-aft rig in its simplicity and the beauty of its aspect
under every angle of vision is, I believe, unapproachable.
A schooner, yawl, or cutter, in charge of a capable man seems
to handle herself as if endowed with the power of reasoning
and the gift of swift execution."* – Joseph Conrad

One calm summer evening in the early 1980s I was on passage from Goderich to Little Current with my wife Jean and friends. Because the winds were virtually none existent, we stayed out on Lake Huron all night, preferring to close the shore and find Fitzwilliam Passage in daylight. Just at dawn I spotted a small white smudge on the southern horizon. Soon it was identified as one of the Toronto Brigantines. As she was making better time, we waited for her to come near. To me, even though she was quite small when compared to such vessels as the St. Lawrence, she was a thing of great beauty and nostalgia.

CHAPTER 16

Schooner Days, Anecdotal Material and Commercial Sail

THE TITLE, "SCHOONER DAYS" was used for 1,303 articles that appeared in the *Toronto Evening Telegram* between 1931 and 1954. All were written by Charles Henry Jeremiah Snider, a great marine historian and storyteller, who eventually became managing editor of the paper in those days. He was born in 1879 at Sherwood, near Maple, Ontario, and died in 1971. Primarily as the result of these articles and his many books, he undoubtedly became the best known and best loved writer on the lake shipping scene, both sail and steam, in Canada's history. He could string a mediocre bit of maritime trivia into an exciting tale of lasting interest, though some say his stories sometimes strayed a bit from history. This was his privilege and should not become a cause for criticism. His writings have formed a major source of material for my chapters on sail after the War of 1812. Though many other books added to my sources, the "Schooner Days" collection was the foremost resource.

Of the schooner days an unknown author has written:

> I can't help feeling lonesome for the old ships that have gone.

For the sight of Huron sunsets and the hours before
the dawn,
And the white sails pullin' stoutly to a warm and
steady draft,
And the smell of roastin' coffee and the watches
must run 'aft.
I'd like to ship off-shore again upon some tidy
barque,
And sing a sailor shantey in the windy starry dark,
Or first a clewed-up tops'l in a black south-easter
roar,
But what's the use of wishing: for them days will
come no more.[1]

The Days of Sail on the Great Lakes from 1815 to 1920

Settlement had begun around the lower lakes prior to the War of
1812. On the cessation of hostilities, rapid colonization commenced
with commercial and agricultural developments at a pace perhaps
unequalled anywhere else at any time. The migration of settlers from
Europe and the Atlantic seaboard was counted in the millions. Lake
navigation played a major role in moving the people, their personal
effects and the produce of their labour. Until the mid-1800s, water
transport was the cheapest and most reliable form of transportation
available. Even after the railways entered the picture, lake transportation continued to grow.

Shipwrights and other artificers from the naval yards were
thrown out of work when the Treaty of Ghent was signed on
Christmas Eve 1814. Many settlers and workers on the British side
returned to their homeland. Many Americans from Sacket's Harbor
and from Lake Erie packed up their tools and went back to families
in Boston, New York and Philadelphia. Others stayed on and settled
as farmers, merchants and tradesmen, sensing the great promises
offered by the new land. However, some saw opportunities north of
the lakes and freely crossed the border to take advantage of situations

as they were presented in the Canadas. Almost every waterfront settlement of any size on both sides of the lower lakes became a shipyard of sorts. Some, such as Toronto, Cleveland, Buffalo and Detroit, grew very rapidly. It was not until the early 1830s that towns further inland, such as Milwaukee and Chicago started to thrive.

Colonists to Canada from the British Isles came to Lake Ontario via the St. Lawrence route, then took a ship to cross the lake from Kingston to Niagara. They then crossed overland by the Niagara Portage Road[2] and re-embarked on Lake Erie. Travel for these early settlers was far from easy. The *Niagara Gleaner* of September 24, 1818, carried this item, "We are sorry to hear that the immigrants from Ireland who passed here about ten days ago on their way to Port Talbot were cast away on board the *Young Phoenix* off Long Point on the South Shore, forty-five miles from Buffalo and narrowly escaped with their lives and lost nearly all their effects. We understand a small vessel was afterwards purchased to carry them to the north side of the Lake." Even Americans from the seaboard found it easier to come up the Hudson River by boat as far as possible, then move down Lake Champlain and the Richelieu River, thence up the St. Lawrence to Lake Ontario. Roads were little more than trails through the woods and despite all the hazards of water travel, it was far more comfortable, faster and less expensive than travelling overland. Travellers need no longer experience the former vexations of land travel. They would be from incessant altercations with landlords with the mutual charges of dishonesty, free from discomforts of dealing with new modes of speech and reckoning money, and free from the breaking down of carriages and wearing out of horses.

Accommodation on board ship was very meagre at first, and comforts essentially non-existent. It was not uncommon on a long trip for a vessel to be storm-bound in the shelter of some headland or otherwise laid up in some uninhabited cove for days. Ships would run out of fresh food. But they always had access to plentiful fresh water. Men ventured ashore to hunt game, or try to acquire some produce from nearby farms, if any were to be found in the vicinity. Frequently, passengers would sleep on deck among the cargo and cattle, for the cabins, such as they were, were often overcrowded and foul with seasickness.

In 1815, a company of merchants at Kingston, Ontario, was formed to finance the construction of a steamship. In October of that year a contract was let to Messrs. Teabout and Chapman, both of whom had been shipwrights at Sacket's Harbor under Henry Eckford. The engines for the new ship came from the Birmingham firm of Boulton and Watt. The new vessel, the *SS Frontenac*, was launched at Finkles Point (near Bath, Ontario) on September 7, 1816, and thus started the steam age on the lakes. The *SS Frontenac* was a resounding success and traded actively until she was burned by vandals at Niagara in 1827.

The Americans were not far behind in adopting steam power for ships, and the *SS Ontario* was built at Sacket's Harbor and launched in March 1817. She was 110 feet long overall; her beam inside guards was 24 feet; the depth of hold was eight feet and her gross tonnage was 240 tons. The following year the *Walk-in-the-Water* was built at Black Rock (near Buffalo) by Noah Brown, the famous shipbuilder of the recent war. She served the Upper Lakes, her principal ports being Buffalo, Erie, Cleveland and Detroit with occasional trips to Michillimackinac. Rates for passage were: Buffalo to Erie, $6.00; to Cleveland, $12.00; and to Detroit, $18.00. She had a short life. On the night of October 30, 1821, she encountered severe weather after leaving Buffalo and started to take on water. It required so much steam to run the pumps that there was not sufficient for the engine. The anchors were dropped, but the leaks became worse and it was decided to run her ashore. At 4:30 a.m. on November l, she struck ground near Port Albino, twelve miles from Buffalo. She fired her gun to summon help but no help was forthcoming. The entire ship's company, passengers and crew, were forced to make their way ashore through the crashing surf. Miraculously, no lives were lost. A new vessel, the *SS Superior* was built, also by Noah Brown, and fitted with the engines salvaged from the *Walk-in-the-Water*. She saw many years of service.

The Erie Canal was first opened in 1826, connecting the lakes with the seaboard via the Hudson River. Captain Samuel Ward of

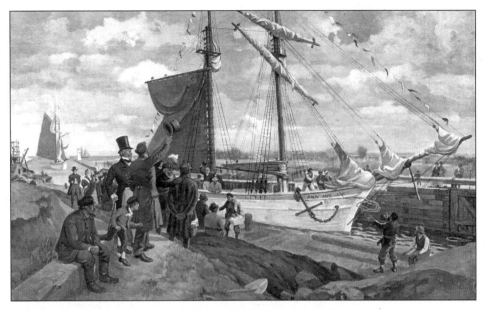

Linking the Great Lakes, J.D. Kelly, artist. *The* Ann and Jane *was the first vessel to pass through the first Welland Canal when it opened on November 27, 1829. This canal linked the Upper Lakes to Lake Ontario and the St. Lawrence.* Courtesy of Confederation Life Insurance Co.

Detroit took a small schooner, the *St. Clair*, through the canal that same year. The ship's masts were lowered at Buffalo and she was towed down the canal to the Hudson where her masts were raised again. This is the same system which pleasure yachts must use today, though they travel under their own power. The *St. Clair* carried the first cargo on any craft from the lakes to salt water without transhipment.

On November 27, 1829, the first Welland Canal was opened, the first passage being made by the Canadian schooner, *Ann and Jane*, of York, from Lake Ontario to Lake Erie. She was followed the same day by the American schooner, *R.H. Broughton*, of Youngstown, Ohio. The *Broughton* had been built on Lake Ontario and thus, for the first time, was able to visit her Port of Registry.

The vessels transiting the canals were towed by teams of horses, or even oxen, often referred to as the "horned breeze." Before long, steam tugs took over the service. The opening of the canals, and their subsequent deepening, helped traffic on the lakes to increase manyfold.

In the period 1800 to 1820, the population of Ohio increased from some 42,000 to 580,000 while that of Michigan increased from 3,757 to 8,765. The arrival of the steamers and the opening of the canals created the greatest spurt of settlement on the Huron and Michigan shores. Some time prior to 1819, the revenue cutter[3] *Fairplay* arrived at Chicago, outside the bar[4] and then proceeded to enter the river. She was the first sailing vessel to anchor in the Chicago River.

A few figures will give some idea of the rate of growth of that area. At the beginning of 1832 only some 150 people lived in the log houses near the little fort on Lake Michigan where the Chicago River entered into it. It had 2,000 inhabitants by the end of the year and 20,000 people had arrived there by boat from the Lower Lakes. By 1837 the population was 8,000. Chicago was a starting point for settlers fanning out over the Illinois lands. But Chicago had no harbour. The schooners had to anchor offshore and passengers and cargo were ferried ashore in small boats and rafts. The sudden storms, which hit that corner of the lake even yet, wrecked many a vessel before she could weigh anchor and get out into open waters. In 1835, some 225 sailing vessels arrived at Chicago, and one year later, nearly 1,000 sailing ships. A similar number of steamships arrivals were recorded at Cleveland.

Steamships quickly took over the passenger trade, primarily because they were much faster and more reliable and they were fitted out with considerable degree of comfort, even grandeur. At the peak of the immigration traffic, the transportation facilities provided by both Canada and the United States were stretched to the limit, far beyond the point of safety. Pioneers, writing of coming west on steamers during the forties and fifties, tell of passengers being packed so closely that it was impossible for the crew to do its work. Every ship bound inland carried from three to five hundred passengers in the cabins and steerage. Many more persons were not unusual. Pioneers tell of going down to the piers in the towns on the west side of Lake Michigan to see steamers that brought up 1,300 to 1,500 passengers.

Business for the ships was highly competitive. Many owners cut prices to the bone to take the traffic away from their competitors, even to the point of crowding on the last few for free. Their early records

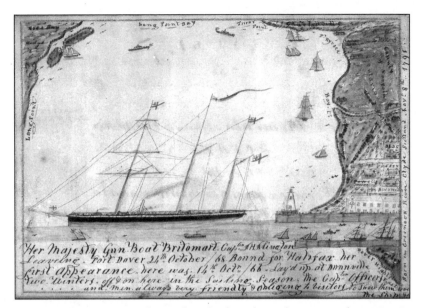

HMS Britomart, *watercolour, ink and coloured pencil on paper, about 6"x 8", Captain Alexander McNeilledge (1791-1874), artist. The script under the painting says: "Her Majesty Gun Boat Britomart Captain H. Alington Leaving Port Dover /68 Bound for Halifax Her first appearance here was 14th Oct'r /66 Layed up at Dunnville two winters off & on here in the Sailing Season. The Captain Officers and men always friendly & obliging to visitors to show them around the ship." On the right side of the painting is the artist's place and date of birth: "Born in Greenock River Clyde Scotland Novr 8th 1791." The Britomart was a Royal Navy gunboat dispatched from Britain to Lake Erie during the Fenian crisis of the mid-1880s. McNeilledge was a very experienced saltwater captain who had traversed the waters of the world, but ultimately settled in the Port Dover area in the 1830s. His most famous contribution to the lake came during the 1840s when he produces charts and maps for navigating Lake Erie. Other McNeilledge artworks, stories and personal artifacts are on display at the Port Dover Harbour Museum.* Courtesy of the Collection of Mary Morrison.

were marred by occasional boiler explosions and fires until the men who tended the engines became sufficiently familiar with the problems of stoking the fires and keeping sufficient water in the boilers.

But, interestingly, the number of sailing vessels continued to increase. The first cargo for these small ships resulted from the fur trade. As the land was cleared, more and more settlers arrived and there was initial need for supplies for the settlements as they were unable, at first, to produce enough food to sustain themselves. The ships transported flour, corn, cheese, whisky and tobacco west from Buffalo, Erie, Cleveland and Sandusky and these cargoes became known as "Ohio fur." In 1830, the schooner *Detroit*, under Captain Robinson, cleared Cayahoga (Cleveland) with a full load, consisting of 91 barrels of flour, 101 barrels of whisky, 63 barrels of pork, 51 barrels of dried fruit, 24 barrels of cider and 16 barrels of beef.

Soon shipments of grain started to move in the opposite direction. The settlers who moved inland in the early days found surprising success with their crops and obtained excellent yields of wheat, oats and barley. In 1836, the brig, *John Kinzie*, loaded up with 3,000 barrels of wheat at Grand River, Michigan, for delivery to Buffalo. The grain was transported in from the farms by wagon, bagged in the dockside warehouses and loaded aboard on the backs of stevedores. In 1838, the steamer, *Great Western*, carried 39 bags of wheat from Chicago to Buffalo. This was the first grain shipment from that port. In October 1839, the brig *Osceola* carried 1,678 bushels of wheat, loading at the Newberry and Dole warehouse on the Chicago River. The grain was brought directly from the farmer's wagons on the inside of the warehouse, hoisted by rope and pulley and "Irish" power, using the muscle of local labour, to the second storey. It later was dumped down a chute to the dockside where it filled four-bushel boxes that were carried aboard and finally dumped into the hold. It certainly was not a masterpiece of labour efficiency!

From these small beginnings, the shipments of grain has grown to fill tens, even hundreds of huge carriers each year, for direct shipment overseas to feed the world's hungry peoples. Nearly every port large enough to handle the ocean-going ships has its own mechanical elevators today. But grain was not the only commercial shipment to leave Chicago, even taking into account the early days of the fur trade. In 1832, George W. Dole built a slaughterhouse there. In April of 1833, he shipped, on the schooner *Napoleon*, 287 barrels of beef, 14 barrels of tallow and 152 hides.

Every conceivable cargo, from the early shipments of furs, fish

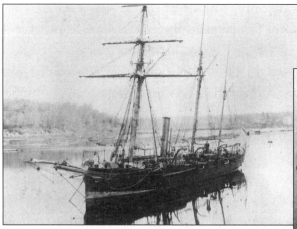

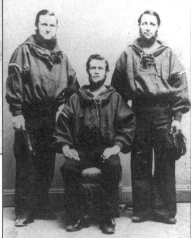

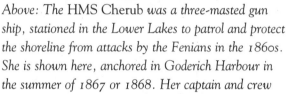

Above: The HMS Cherub *was a three-masted gun ship, stationed in the Lower Lakes to patrol and protect the shoreline from attacks by the Fenians in the 1860s. She is shown here, anchored in Goderich Harbour in the summer of 1867 or 1868. Her captain and crew were reputed to enjoy an ongoing fete of social activities, often being the guests of honour at the homes of distinguished residents. They would host gala events designed to impress friends and acquaintances with the presence of the naval officers. The* Cherub *was an early steam-assisted sailing vessel, Her sister ship, the* HMS Prince Alfred *often travelled in tandem with her. Right: Members of the crew of the* Cherub *posing for a formal photograph.* Both photos courtesy of the Huron County Museum.

and grain, through ore and stone, copper, iron and limestone, lumber, manufactured articles, farm machinery, furniture and much, much more, was carried by sail in the early days.

Gradually, bulk carriers took over the trade for high volume cargo, but sail continued to carry the package goods. In 1843, the schooner *Dolphin* passed down the Ohio Canal from Cleveland to New Orleans with a load of whitefish. In 1844, the brigantine *Pacific* took a cargo of wheat and flour from Toronto to Liverpool. In 1849, the St. Lawrence canals were improved to permit the passage of vessels with a nine-foot draft. The barque *Eureka* sailed all the way from Cleveland around Cape Horn to San Francisco, with 59 passengers bound for the gold fields of California.

All the early steamships on the lakes were sidewheelers. It was not until 1841 that the first propeller-driven vessel was launched, the *SS Vandalia*, built at Oswego, New York. Not only was she the first propeller-driven vessel on the lakes, but the first commercially-operated propeller vessel in the world, and the first steam vessel with her machinery aft of amidships.

Before this time, several schooners had been hauled out below the rapids, put on skids or rollers and dragged overland up to Lake Superior. There they were relaunched and used as traders among the communities around the south and west shores of the lake. The first of these was the 55-ton *Algonquin*, in 1839. Generally, this overland trip would be done in winter when the ground was frozen and could support the great weight.

Among the many sailing vessels to make this overland passage from the lower lakes were the *Chippewa*, *Florence*, *Swallow*, *Merchant*, *Uncle Tom*, and the *Fur Trader*. One steamer, the propeller vessel, *Independence*, of 260 tons, made this passage with the others, all in the season 1845-46. The schooners ranged in tonnage from twenty to one hundred and ten tons. In subsequent years, more and larger ships crossed overland, the passage taking many weeks of very slow transit, the motive power being horses and capstan.

In 1850, the first propeller vessel to leave the lakes, the 400-ton *Ontario*, set out from Buffalo for San Francisco. That same year, the *Sophia* of Kingston, a topsail schooner sailed from her home port to Liverpool and was sold there. Many vessels were built on the Great Lakes for the British market after this transaction. In 1855, the brig *Columbia* brought the first load of Lake Superior iron ore through the Sault Canal to the port of Cleveland.

In 1865, the 200-ton brig *Sea Gull* sailed from Toronto to Durban, South Africa, and got back before freeze-up the same year. She carried a cargo of farm machinery, wagons, buggies and flour for farms in the interior. She never left the lakes again.

The heyday of sail on the lakes would be reached around 1870 when some 2,000 sailing ships were on the lists. Eighty percent of them were schooners. Barques and brigs made up the balance. Soon after this, commercial sail started to dwindle as steam bulk-carriers were taking over the trade.

COMMERCIAL SAIL ON THE LAKES

Every coastal town of any size had one shipyard or more. There was a continual desire to build bigger and better ships, but the limitations of the canals and the shallow draft of both canals and harbour entrances put severe restrictions on the size of vessels. In general, the early ships were very small by today's standards, in fact, many were smaller than some of the pleasure yachts that ply the same waters today.

One cannot generalize and say that all the craft were well-designed and skillfully built – nor vice versa. In general, the ships were built as well as necessary for the purpose, or as well as the owner could afford. Pride sometimes required the finest that money could buy, yet at other times lack of funds would necessitate a vessel somewhat less pretentious than perhaps it should have been for the trade. Individual owners would, at times, build in their own ideas of what a ship should be like.

Sometimes this course of action produced improvements, but at other times the result was to construct a vessel that was extremely "crank." This term refers to a vessel that was generally hard to steer and perhaps had a habit of making the decision of which way to go rather than leaving that decision to the man at the wheel. An example of such poor design was the *Royal Oak*, built at Kingston in 1852, as a 175-ton schooner. She was rebuilt at Adolphustown in 1884, and renamed the *Fabiola* at that time. This may occasioned the beginning of her steering troubles, "The *Fabiola* was known as a very peculiar vessel to steer. To look at her hull when in dry dock, she was considered a very nice model, especially aft, where she had a long, clean run." Someone remarked, "She must steer like a yacht!"

But not so! According to Snider, "She was a very uneasy ship, not heavy to steer, but you never could tell what she would do. If she was 'coming up' or 'going off' and you gave her enough wheel to check her you would expect her to swing back the opposite way, but not always so, for she was as apt to start right on, up or off, as the case might be. Her compass was rather slow to start, especially when there was no sea to rock it. As she would start, up or off, you would hear a roar of water around one quarter or the other quarter as she raced around. If below at meals in calm weather we could hear it in the cabin, and knew the problem the man at the wheel was having. The helmsman kept a whittled stick to poke the compass in the binnacle and make it respond."[5]

One must remember too, that there was a continual evolvement in hull and rig and generally in new technology for ship construction. Initially, hulls needed to be very shallow draft in order to navigate rivers and cross the sandbars at the entrance to harbours. Once the canals were opened, they dictated the maximum draft and the overall dimensions of the vessels, much as they still do today.

The trimness and beauty of the ships built at Kingston and at Sacket's at the end of the war, was rarely duplicated in the early commercial vessels built elsewhere. From the outset, military requirements to the contrary, the fore-and-aft rig was preferred on the lakes.[6]

Captain Bradley, in a letter to Boscawen (both were part of the British army who occupied Oswego in 1755) dated September 15, 1755, wrote, "I acquainted you in my letter of the 21st August, that His Excellency, Major General Shirley, etc., had order'd the *Ontario* to be made a sloop…. She sails extremely well and is, in every respect a much better vessel than the SCHOONER I command. Upon my return here on the 13th and acquainting Major General Shirley how well the Sloop behaved, we came to the resolution to alter the *Oswego* as soon as the extended Expedition is over."[7]

So we have yet another *Oswego*, at least the third to share that name in marine history.[8] What was needed was a rig that provided ample sail area for running before steadily favourable winds on down-lake passages, and, at the same time, sails that could be easily handled in entering or leaving restricted harbours, or for tacking and beating off a lee shore in a hurry without too much fuss.

In further complaint, Captain Bradley wrote to Cleveland on September 26, 1756, "…on the same day in running into Oswego, was taken with a violent Thunder Squall, close to the Harbor, which after my getting through the Narrows, not being able to carry Sail, drove me ashore on the East Side of the Harbor, which obliged me to get my guns and part of my Ballast out to get her (the brig) off again." Bradley obviously wished to underscore his point that a change in rig was imperative.

Naval vessels were built for mobility and fighting ability. There was generally little restriction to the number of crew available. Commercial vessels, on the other hand, were more concerned with cargo-carrying capacity, economy of initial cost and economy of operations. The smaller the crew required to handle a vessel, the better. Usually the commercial vessels would carry one-fourth, or even less, crew than that of a naval vessel of the same size.

The three-masted square rig of the naval vessels gave an added security for, should one mast be shot away, the vessel could still manoeuvre well with the remaining two. The square rig sails presented smaller targets and more numerous units than the fore-and-after. A broadside against a fore-and-after could well damage boom or gaff, making all sail attached to that mast useless. The square riggers, in spite of being less easily managed than a fore-and-after, gave a very good account of themselves in the War of 1812. However, the large ships-of-the line, that had begun to appear towards the end of the war were really impractical on such a small body of water as Lake Ontario.

For commerce, the square rigger was totally impractical and uneconomic. However, to achieve better speeds down wind some compromise was necessary and most of the fore-and-afters had square sails on the foremast. A few were built with square sails on both the foremast and mainmast, and a very few were ship-rigged with square sails on all three masts.

To assist in the identification of the different classes of craft as discussed here, some definitions are given here to provide some clarification and relate to the locale and the era. A schooner was a two-masted vessel whose aftermast, which was the mainmast, consisted of a lower mast and topmast (the combination being taller than the foremast) and carried a gaff mainsail, gaff topsail and staysail. The rig of the foremast varied and these variations gave rise to different names. If the whole foremast was fully rigged, the vessel was called either a hermaphrodite brig or brigantine or simply a brig. When the foremast carried a gaff on the lower, and a square sail on the topmast, she was called a topsail schooner. Square sails on the topmast of both masts did not change the name; she was still a schooner and the *Nancy* was a very pretty example of such a vessel.

If there were no square sails the name applied was fore-and-after schooner. If three masts, with no square sails, she was a three-and-after, at least in some parts of the lakes. If square sails were used on the fore-topmast, she was a barquentine or barque or simply a bark. Some were built with four masts and one had five, as did the *David Dows* of Toledo.

These are the names that appear to have been applied in the majority of cases to lake vessels, but sailors' language is not always precise. The vessels, which combined the fore-and-aft rig with the square rig, proved to be admirably suited to lake conditions, easily handled and capable of a fair turn of speed, even when heavily loaded. Whether the brigs and barks actually originated on the lakes is doubtful, however they did achieve popularity here somewhat earlier than in salt water. Schooners and brigs were the most common types of rigs.

At the beginning of the second half of the 19th century, according to James Mills, there were, in all the lakes, 95 steamboats, 45 propellers, five barques, 93 brigs, 548 schooners and 128 sloops and scows. The aggregate tonnage was 153,454 tons.[9]

Although for many years the need continued for shallow draft vessels in order to navigate the canals and cross the harbour bars, centreboards were not applied to large vessels until the middle of the century. In Manitowac, Wisconsin, in 1852, a builder by the name of William Bates, laid down a clipper-bowed brigantine equipped with a huge centreboard, some 10 feet by 12 feet below the keel. The *Challenge* is reported to be the first such type and proved to be exceptionally fast, easily achieving thirteen knots.[10] The *Clipper City* and the *Manitowac* followed her. The style rapidly became the standard for small vessels on the lakes. Plans for the *Challenge* were taken to Paris by a French naval constructor as an example of a clipper centreboard vessel. They were published in France and have provided us with some design details and lines. However, very few draughts are available with lines for early Great Lakes vessels. Not content with one centreboard, some builders tried to apply two and three boards to their designs. Such features were not common, except in the case of some of the sailing scows, which had as many as four boards.

The rig of most of the lake schooners was not essentially different from that of ocean-going ships of the same style, except in respect to mast height. On the ocean, typically, all masts were of equal height. On the lakes, it was customary for the foremast, and mizzen if there was one, to be slightly shorter than the main mast.

Up to about 1820, many of the vessels would draw up, or brail their sails but this changed to the system of furling by lowering the gaffs. Brailing continued to a lesser extent, however, and the *Rastus C. Corning* of Buffalo used this system up to 1890. Around 1870, a triangular topsail (or raffee) came into vogue. It was frequently accompanied by an extra large square sail known as a runner. The runner was found on ocean ships as well but the raffee never seemed to be used on these ocean-going vessels. There were many other variations as time went on, such as the Grand Haven rig, described later, in connection with timber droghers.

In general, the large sail craft of the lakes used a flat, broad transom, and were built for practical use rather than for beauty. The stone hookers and those built for the sand trade and similar purposes were little more than scows rigged with sails, albeit the sail plan was generally a close copy of the rig used on their prouder sisters.

The canallers, those vessels that were built especially for use in the canals of the early days, were designed to fit into the locks, just, and with little or no room to spare. Even the bowsprit had to be especially designed and was either very short, very steeply steeved, or capable of being hauled inboard for passage in the locks. The canallers were blunt-bowed, flat-sided vessels, little better than floating boxes with sails and centreboards.

Some lake vessels were exceptionally well-built and furnished. They carried elaborately carved figureheads and were trimmed with delicate filigree work. They showed beautiful, clean lines and fancy carving. Magnificent name boards decorated their transoms.

The five-masted *David Dows* of Toledo, built in 1881 (275 feet long), was the largest schooner anywhere at the time. Her planking at the turn of the bilge was half-a-foot thick, and she had over 70,000 yards of canvas and two centreboards. She sported a figurehead representing a dragon. She may have been too large a vessel to be practical, for she was involved in two collisions and experienced the loss of several seamen. She then was converted to a tow barge but only lasted until November 1889, when she sank near Chicago. She was the longest sailing ship ever built on the lakes but not the largest when displacement is taken into account. That record remains with the *St. Lawrence*.

By all accounts, one of the prettiest ships on the lakes was the *Minnedosa*, 225 feet long, 36-foot beam, 18-foot hold and 1,200 tons displacement. She was built at Kingston in 1890 for the grain trade. She worked from the head of the lakes to the St. Lawrence River. Like the *David Dows*, she was built especially strong. Her floor frames, crossing her bottom, were 18" deep and 18" wide, each one as heavy as an average vessel's keel or keelson, and they were only five inches apart. There were over a hundred of these massive frames. A sheer-strake of 5/8" steel, 18" deep, ran around her outside at deck level. Inside her, for extra strength, were diagonal steel straps, forming diamond shapes some five feet across.

One unnamed reporter at the time has written, "She had a very handsome stern, rounded to a perfect ellipse. Her cutwater knee and the figurehead were as beautiful as any yacht's or clipper ship's; in fact, the finest ever shown on freshwater. It was a life-size, half-length figure of Ceres, Greek goddess of harvest, with a cornucopia inverted behind her, out of which poured the bounty of corn and wheat, running along the cheek knees in a beautiful scroll. At each end of the headrails, was a Canadian beaver, with a maple branch in his mouth. Between the beavers was the name Minnedosa in gilt letters. The catheads for the anchors each bore a cat's head, carved in relief and painted to the life. The figureheads and trailboards use $1,000 worth

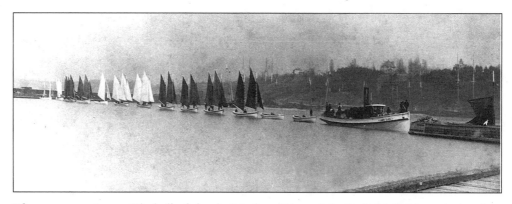

The steam tug, James Clark *(built by the Marlton Shipyards in Goderich Harbour during the 1870s), is hauling the Goderich-based fishing fleet out to the fishing grounds, a daily task for the tug. By the mid-1880s catches had fallen off in the southern Lake Huron area and the fleet was now being towed north to fishing grounds near the mouth of the Saugeen River. The Huron-Signal of Goderich published the photo on August 28, 1886, and attributed the "staged" photo to R.R. Sallows. The tug boat captain was identified as Captain Ed McGregor. "The fish boats in tow were;* Pearl Elizabeth, *Craig & Patterson;* Wave, *James Sutherland;* Heather Belle, *Alex and Thos. Craigie;* Maple Leaf, *John Craigie;* Wm Saunders, *James Clark, John Bain;* Flying Cloud, *Daniel McKay;* Goderich Belle, *McDonald Bros.;* Foam, *James Inkster;* Peruvian, *Dan Matheson;* Alaska, *James Clark;* Parisian, *Jas. Clark... ."* Courtesy of the Huron County Museum.

of work and gold leaf. N. Henderson of Kingston, a contemporary artist in oils, was the designer and supervisor of the decoration; Louis Gourdier was the carver. The vessel herself was satiny black from stem to stern, with white cabin and large white deck-forecastle, a novelty on the lakes. Her mastheads were black. The monotony of 200 feet of unbroken bulwarks was relieved by three panels picked out in yellow beading. She carried four top-masts."

Just at what time towing started is not clear, but steam tugs were used early on to haul the craft through the Detroit and St. Clair rivers, the St. Mary's River and in and out of harbours. Before long, it was only natural that they should be used for long hauls when the wind was adverse, and the idea proved economically sound. Soon it became quite common for some of the old schooners, brigs and barques to have their masts cut down and to be towed the length of the lakes. They would carry, in addition to their cargo, sufficient wood to stoke the boilers of the steam tugs. The sails would be used if the winds were favourable and could add any power to the passage. Should a towed vessel be separated from her tug in a heavy storm, her chance of survival was very slim with her reduced rig.

In 1869, John Brandt Mansfield provides us with another list of vessels in use: 126 steamers, 140 propellers, 240 tugs, 175 barques, 50 brigs, 904 schooners, plus countless small sloops, scows and ketches.[11] As noted earlier, the peak number on the lakes is variously reported to exceed 2,000 sail vessels. Sadly, the pinnacle for the age of sail had now passed. Steam had now assumed the primary motive role. The last sailing ships had been built, and as they wore out, were lost or converted to barges, they were no longer being replaced. Walter Havighurst says the *Lucie A. Simpson*, built at Manitowac in 1875, and wrecked near Sturgeon Bay in 1929, was the last of the large sailing ships.[12]

Life for the sailor in the early days was extremely hard and dangerous but full of adventure and colour. The crews came to the lakes from all the countries of Europe plus the coastal communities of Canada and the United States. They formed a community of nations on the lakes and were attracted by the higher wages and by the fact that trips were shorter with more time in port. Whether the cargo was grain or iron ore, or whatever, the sailors frequently had the added job of working as their own stevedores, loading and unloading the cargo. Fare was plain: salt pork or beef, fish, hard bread, potatoes, beans, corn and plenty of whisky (half a pint per man per day). In town, the crew caroused and drank their way around the waterfront dives, being no different from seamen of their day elsewhere in the world.

Although a fore-and-after was not as dangerous, nor as difficult as the square-riggers of comparable size, the sailors were forced to contend with severe and sudden storms, ships top-heavy with ice, and similar hazards. Many lost their lives or were seriously injured in accidents, fires, collisions, shipwrecks and so on. Many drowned or were frozen to death. There were no rules concerning safety. There was no compensation for injury or death. No board, union or government agency looked after their welfare.

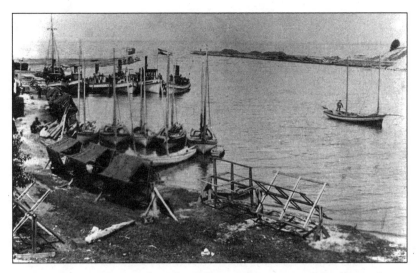

Southampton, at the mouth of the Saugeen River, may well have been the earliest fishing port established along the Canadian shore of Lake Huron. Sailing activity, identified through archaeological studies, was present during the late 1700s. In this pre-1883 photo, the fleet of fishing vessels and tugs is shown. The date of the photo precedes the construction of the outer range light (built in 1883 and which would be seen in the background following that date), but it certainly is after the construction of the Chantry Island Light (c.1850). The man standing in the small sailboat, mid-river, is Lance Bellmore. In the mid-left of the photo, there are two people seated. They are Murdock Matheson and Mrs. Finley MacLennan, formerly Mrs. (George) Margaret MacAulay. George MacAulay drowned off the Fishing Islands, November 2, 1865, in a late fall storm. The Mathesons, MacLennans and MacAulays were well-known waterfront names in the Southampton commu-nity for generations. Courtesy of Don Morton of Seaforth, Ontario.

Not until 1909, did the Lake Carriers' Association initiate a Welfare Plan to pay meagre death benefits to the relatives of regis-tered seamen who had died in every manner of calamity on the lakes. While the number of payments was but 21 in 1912, the total of 123 was reached in 1913 after the terrible "Great Storm" of November that year. Of the recorded 153 lives lost, most were voluntary mem-bers of the Welfare Plan. A total of $17,825 was paid in death bene-fits, ranging from $75 for the loss of a porter, an ordinary seaman or a 2nd cook, and up to $500 for a ship's master.[13]

Finally, embarrassed that no compensation could be paid by the Ontario government of the day, Premier Sir James Pliny Whitney's Conservative government passed a new Workmen's Compensation Act. It would, according to Opposition Leader N.C. Rowell, permit Ontario to catch up as, "…in poor backward Russia … in Spain… in Australia, … New Zealand, … South Africa," and in several Canadian Provinces. "Ontario is the one large country under the British flag that has not such an act," he declared.[14] In addition, following major catastrophes on the lakes, the Carriers' Association and local communities often set up Lakes Disaster Funds, for which the names of contributors were listed in the local newspapers.[15]

Wages in 1818 were $15 per month for ordinary seamen, $25 to $30 for mates and $40 to $50 for masters. By 1836 these had risen to $18 to $35 for seamen, stewards and engineers, $36 to $40 for first mates, and captains received $600 to $800 for the entire season. By 1860, the seaman's wages had risen to $2 per day.

C.J.N. Snider spent some time on ships on the lakes before and between his writing activities. He has written of life in the forecastle of a couple of schooners in the last days of sail. In addition to his very informed manner of writing about the maritime life, he also expressed strong feelings about the use of proper, seagoing pronunciation in the spoken word. For example, he stressed that the proper utterance "folksel," "forksel," "fawksel," must be used, but never "forecastle," as the word was actually spelled. He offered a superb description of the *Oliver Mowat*, a three-masted schooner with a long career on the lakes. She offered a great "fo'c's'l":

> Her forecastle had four bunks each side, one above the other, and aft of them two great lockers containing chain. These served as benches. The berths were fitted with straw mattresses and with bunk boards, and were provided with patch quilts and pillows. Spare berths were filled with coils of rope, spare blocks and gear.
>
> All was painted either buff or white or pale blue. There was a pot-bellied, little Quebec heater, and in

front of it a square box, filled with sawdust, called the spit-kid. And see that you hit it every time, young fellow, for the man who misses has to clean up.

This requirement was an absolute, the "nonpareil" of schooner days.

The worst "fo'c's'l" he ever visited, and he declines the name of the vessel, was, he says:

>...typical of the product of owner's niggardliness, master's indifference, and sailors' laziness. It was called the bear pit. So dark you couldn't see into it by day or night without a lantern. The lamp was rusty and dirty and gave very little light. The wretched hole had never been painted. Wood was darkened and stained with coal dust, soot, grain dust and iron ore. Stained with spray and rain through the open scuttle, sweat of an unventilated enclosure and seepage of the five Great Lakes through deck and sides and the return of the bilgewater from the pumps which could not escape through the scuppers. The bunks were filled with mouldy straw covered with sacks and mildewed bedding. The stove was a raw, red, rusted, shell of oft-burned iron. The place was alive with bed-bugs. Rat holes plugged with broken necks of whiskey bottles served as scuppers. Thank goodness we never had to eat in the forecastle. Lake sailors dined where the mate dined, at the cabin table, and of the same fare. The cabin was always clean or the cook walked the plank.

Of the *Adriadne* he says, "Each bunk edge or deck beam was serrated with a series of notches. They were the tally sheets of departed mariners, who kept their own 'time' by cutting a notch for each day. Another day, another dollar. The notch cutting was rarely disputed." He went on to say, "Cooking the books could not be practised with much success, as the pay-offs [pay days] came too frequently."

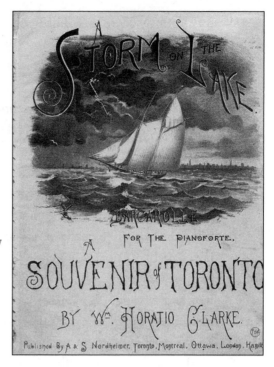

The image comprises an 1884 engraving of the yacht, Oriole, by J.D. Kelly, as shown on the cover of "A Storm on the Lake," with piano music composed by William Horatio Clarke. The gaff-rigged schooner has encountered a sudden storm on Lake Ontario. The piano music is available from the Sheet Music from Canada's Past Collection in the Digital Library of Canada at the National Library of Canada. Courtesy of Walter Lewis, Maritime History of the Great Lakes webmaster.

It was the custom for the sailors to sing as they worked, a tradition brought to the lakes from the saltwater ships. The voyageurs had always sung ballads or shanties in previous centuries as they paddled the lakes and rivers from dawn to sundown. Good singers got a bonus, and a man with some small talent with fiddle, fife or accordion was always in demand. The music provided a rhythm for working the capstan or hauling the lines. It provided a welcome diversion in off-hours, and helped to alleviate the boredom of long passages. There is something arousing about the old sea shanties. They stir feelings inside one's soul, in a manner for which it is hard to account. Personally I have never heard the old shanties sung by seamen in their element. However, I have had the pleasure of several meetings, over a period of some years, with an assembly of men of like interest, who call themselves The Shellbacks and whose regular weekly luncheons in Toronto are frequently enlivened with a gam of sorts about the old days and a few rousing sea shanties.

There are stories about Snider visiting local taverns frequented by the local tars, just to gather stories, and the words to some of the shanty songs. In Goderich, at the Bedford Hotel, the story is told by retired mariner Captain A. Roy Munday, of Snider trying to purchase the words to the shanty, "Scribbler Murphy," from one Malcolm Graham, another local mariner. Of course, Graham refused. But, as the evening wore on, and as the effect of the refreshments softened the sometimes cantankerous environment, the words began to flow, "Scribbler Murphy had a schooner named the *Mohawk*, And he'd scrub her down whenever he left the dock...." And Snider achieved his pursuit without buying a round.

Most times the shanty songs would begin: "Come all ye true born shanty boys, whoever that ye be, I would have you pay attention and listen unto me."

CHARTS, LIGHTHOUSES AND OTHER AIDS

Charts and other aids to navigation were either totally non-existent or extremely limited. The first lighthouse on the lakes was a stone tower, some 45 feet high at Gibraltar Point, off York, in 1804. It functioned all through the War of 1812, guiding friend and foe for safer passage. The first on the Lower Lakes were at Buffalo and at Erie in 1818; and at Presque Isle, Michigan, in 1819; at Cleveland in 1820; at the Lake Huron entrance to the St. Clair River in 1825; and at Chicago in 1832. The first on Lake Superior was at Whitefish Point in 1847.

To whatever degree these lights may have helped the master or the pilot, no buoyage system was in use for a great many years. Captains were expected to make and update their own charts from whatever information was available, and to compare notes with one another for mutual safety. Frequently, the first discovery of a previously unknown hazard ended in disaster. Many a shoal, rock or reef, as shown on our modern charts, are named after the vessel that was the first to encounter them.

The first survey of the lakes, at least on the Canadian side, was done by Captain Gother Mann of the British Army in 1788. He spent most of his time in Lake Huron and Georgian Bay and only charted as far west as Sault Ste. Marie. It has been suggested, but not verified, that he used the schooner *Dunmore* of Detroit. He explored and charted many coves and harbours for the first time. His party discovered heavy, masonry ruins on an island of Nottawasaga Bay. These were portions of the Jesuit Mission station of 1649, abandoned and unseen by the white man for 139 years. The remains of some parts of the stone walls lay largely forgotten on what is now known as Christian Island, today a tourist stop for boat tours.

"A great solitude, little known or frequented except by some Indians," was Mann's description of Georgian Bay.[16] Many of us who cruise the remote channels today in our pleasure yachts can still find inlets and coves where the solitude has little changed. The importance of survey work, especially in these isolated areas, cannot be underestimated.

On the American side, apart from the Boundary Commission of 1818, little surveying was done until 1841, when a survey was commissioned by the US Congress. It took some 40 years to complete and has been updated almost constantly ever since. A member of the British contingent of the commission, Dr. John J. Bigsby, left us an extensive diary of his travels, which make intriguing reading today. His book, *Shoe and Canoe, or, Pictures of Travel in the Canadas*, was printed in London in 1850.

Another diary, that of Major Joseph Delaphield of the American survey team, was not published until 1943 and is less well known but of similar interest in spite of its long title, *The Unfortified Boundary – A Diary of the First Survey of the Canadian Boundary Line from St. Regis to the Lake of the Woods by Articles Major Joseph Delaphield, American Agent Under VI and VII of the Treaty of Ghent*. The editors, Robert McElroy and Thomas Riggs of New York, must have struggled with the title in 1943.

Early charting extended only to a maximum depth of 18 feet, but as ships became larger and deeper, it was necessary to resurvey to 20 feet. On this survey, new hazards were found that undoubtedly had caused wreckings and total losses before these obstacles were charted. The first three of the American charts appeared in 1852. Today, the availability numbers well into the hundreds, and charts of every description can easily be downloaded from internet sources for use on computers, or can be printed to order.

Charting information has become so sophisticated today, that new electronic navigation charts, or ENCs, used on computers, add more information as the user zooms in for a closer look. In one isolated location near Drummond Island, for example, even the long-abandoned individual pilings on an old dock can be seen on the large scale electronic images. Satellite photography is sometimes overlaid, or can be viewed side-by-side, to corroborate ship location. And, of course, with the precise tracking information available from global positioning systems, or GPS, navigators not only know their exact location within a few feet, but also can watch their vessel proceed through treacherous waters on a computer monitor or chart-plotter screen.

Some of the basic programs, available even to pleasure boaters, include as standard options, audible alarms, should one venture into shallow waters, or approach obstacles. The new technology is so overwhelming. The chartware even talks to the user, providing instructions and directions. However, it must be noted, and even underscored, that there is no replacement for human involvement. The need to employ old-fashioned charting skills, along with astute observation techniques, combined with careful decision making taken to supplement these wonderful aids cannot be over emphasized. Shorelines change, bottom sands shift with storms and currents – and satellites sometimes fail.

Captain William Fitzwilliam Owen was appointed chief hydrographer for the lakes by the British in 1815. He was already a renowned explorer and cartographer having spent many years in this work in the Indian Ocean and the East Indies. He had joined the British navy in 1788 at the age of 14. His chief assistants in 1815 were Thomas Emeric Vidal and John Harris, Master, RN. The vessel they used was the schooner *Huron*.

Henry Wolsey Bayfield was only 20 years of age when he was posted to the lake survey in September 1816. He continued as chief hydrographer (he replaced Owen one year later) on the Great Lakes until 1825 and left excellent charts, many of which form the basis for charts which are still in use today. The survey lasted nine years and was long and arduous work. But it was of such a calibre that every man who followed in Bayfield's footsteps in the survey field has admired his work. Captain J.G. Boulton, who at a later date resurveyed some of the same waters, has said of him, "The Admiralty Survey Service has produced good men from Captain Cook onwards, but I doubt whether the British navy has ever produced so gifted and zealous a surveyor as Bayfield."[17] Survey work continued all winter long, holes being chopped through the ice to sound and determine depths. The hardships of the work were considerable, but Bayfield does not appear to have been affected. He lived to be 90 years of age, attained the rank of admiral and died at his home in Prince Edward Island.

Owen is commemorated by the naming of Owen Sound, both the city and the sound. Fitzwilliam Island sits at the entrance to Georgian Bay with Owen Channel to the north and Fitzwilliam Channel to the south of it, between Fitzwilliam and Yeo islands. Bayfield has the village on the Huron shore named after him, plus a reef, a sound and a village on the Superior shore of Wisconsin, another in New Brunswick and an island in Quebec. He honoured members of his family by naming islands at the entrance to Bayfield Sound after them, thus: Henry, for his father; Fanny, for his mother; and Gertrude, for his daughter. A large bay in the same sound is named after his wife, Elizabeth. Close by this area to the north of Manitoulin Island is Vidal Bay, and a lake adjoining Bayfield Sound bears the name, Wolsey. Harris Island and Bayfield Reef guard the passage into Lansdowne Channel, between Centre and Badgeley islands. The early cartographers made sure they would not be forgotten and it adds something of the pleasure of our cruising when we know where the names originate.

It is challenging to visualize the size of this job. The water area of the lakes is some 96,000 square miles with approximately two-thirds of it lying in the United States. The length of the shoreline is over 8,000 miles, of which some 4,700 miles are American, and 3,300 miles comprise Canadian shoreline. Compare this with the entire

American coastline on the Atlantic, Pacific and Mexican waters, excluding Alaska and the Islands, which total only about 5,000 miles.

THE SEAMAN'S LIFE

Nothing can better portray the problems, risks and life styles of the early men of the lakes, than to recount a few anecdotes from the extensive articles of noted marine historian C.H.J. Snider:

> The *Hercules* has the honour of being the first ship-wreck to occur near Chicago. It happened in October 1818. The wreck was found several days late by a band of Natives, but the bodies could not be identified as they had been severely "gnawed by bears and wolves.
>
> The 300-ton schooner, *Annie M. Foster* of Prince Edward was "run down one night in the middle of Lake Ontario by the Dr. Warner's Safe Cure man of Rochester in a $100,000 steam yacht. Afterwards he would never venture into Canadian ports, or if he could avoid it, into Canadian waters. Vengeance came when the yacht went aground in the Batteau Channel near Horseshoe Island. The tugs were sent for and the sheriff arrived on one with a writ.
>
> The *Bonnie Doon* was a small, two-masted schooner of 200 tons that was wrecked on Bois Blanc Island in a late November gale in 1869. Her crew started to walk to Escanaba, 225 miles away, after reaching the Michigan shore. Six of them got there in great distress. The others froze to death. In June of 1868, the American barque, *Cortland*, built in Sheboygan in 1867, of 676 tons, collided with the steamer, *Morning Star*, between Point Pelee and Cleveland. Ten from the barque and 32 from the steamer were drowned.
>
> On August 9, 1841, the barque, *Erie*, was rocked by a tremendous explosion just 33 miles from Chicago.

She was carrying a load of immigrants. All on board perished in the explosion and the fire that followed.

The *Fortune* was struck by lightning on Lake Erie on May 1, 1862, while making canvas after a heavy thunder squall. A bolt of lightning killed both mates who were working the halliards near the base of the mast.

The schooner *Adirondack* cleared from Chicago for Buffalo on October 17, 1866. Five days later, off the Highlands of Au Sable, in Lake Huron, she was struck by a squall and hove down, her cargo of wheat shifting, leaving her on her beams ends. After losing her yawl boat and cutting away both masts, she drifted with one side of her deck under water. On November 2, the barque *Sunnyside* passed and rescued the men who had lived far nine days on the hulk, eating only boiled wheat.

Then *Anne Bellchambers* was a small schooner used for hauling cordwood on Lake Ontario when, on November 25, 1875, she was unable to enter the Eastern Gap at Toronto and had to anchor offshore. The skipper and son, a lad of fifteen, were forced to take to the rigging as waves were sweeping the deck and the vessel became waterlogged. Only the cordwood in the hold kept her afloat. At daybreak, a rescue boat came out, cut father and son from the rigging where they were encased in ice. The boy was dead and his father kept repeating unceasingly, 'It won't be long now, Joe. Soon it will be daylight and they'll see us.' It was thus he tried to comfort his son all through the black November night.

From the Barrie, Ontario, paper of November 17, 1858, "Mutiny. Three men belonging to the barque, *Grace Greenwood*, named Kirkwood, Smith and Elliott, were placed in our jail Tuesday morn by Chief Constable Birnie. It appears these men were highly

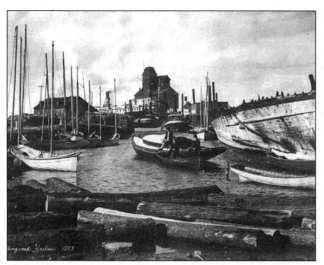

By 1883 Collingwood Harbour was a bustling centre of industry. With the coming of the Ontario, Simcoe and Huron Railway in 1857, the harbour had become an important shipping point for ship repairs. On May 24, 1883, the shipbuilding activities became known as the Collingwood Shipyards, which persisted until 1986. In the photograph, note the presence of the small pleasure craft, albeit a non-sailing, motorized vessel. Photo from a poster in the collection of R. Graham MacDonald. Courtesy of Paul Carroll.

intoxicated when the vessel put to sea from Collingwood on Friday last, and finding out that the captain intended putting into the Severn for lumber, they considered it a breach of contract and refused to work the vessel unless paid extra. During the dispute at sea, these men threatened the life of the captain and others of the crew who ventured to work and, in consequence the vessel was thrown on her beam ends by the heavy winds then prevailing. The vessel was again brought into Collingwood, the men arrested and examined before the magistrate, and were sentenced to 30 days imprisonment."

The *Ann Harkley* was a small schooner from Owen Sound that had, for mate, one John McDuff or "Sailor John," of Simcoe County. Sailor John brought the *Ann Harkley* into Collingwood on October 31, 1866, and entered a "protest." He had left his captain and owner ashore somewhere. The vessel had left Sarnia on October 8, with 170 barrels of whisky and 50 barrels of coal oil. She had heavy weather on Lake Huron and got aground several times before reaching Collingwood. In those days, every sailor wore a gimlet (a small bore) and was expert at driving up a cask-hoop, boring a gimlet hole where the hoop had been, tapping the cask, and driving the hoop back over the plugged hole. Consequently, leakage in a cargo of whisky was frequently large.

The *Magellan* was a canaller built in St. Catharines in 1873. In November 1877, she claimed her turn at the elevator in Chicago in spite of the effort of the master of the steam barge, M. W. Head, to block her. She got her load of corn and sailed out. Ratsy Ratcliffe, the master of the Head vowed vengeance as he considered the other vessel to have claimed his place in line, and swore that, sooner or later, he would put the Magellan on a lee shore, even if he had to do it with the Head's stem. This was a formidable oak timber, iron-shod and project-ing full twenty inches beyond the rabbet. Nosing into a northeaster, the Head failed to make progress, and Captain "Ratsy," in the throes of delirium tremens after drowning his rage, decided to stand in for the shelter of Long Shoal, near Manitowac. His engineer and first mate overpowered him when he became completely maniacal, and contin-ued the barge's course for the intended anchorage. On reaching it, they found a number of lake vessels, steam and sail, already sheltering in the lee of the shoal, with the Wisconsin shore to leeward of them.

As they prepared to anchor, "Ratsy" broke loose from his berth, and, rushing to the wheelhouse, cried, "There she is, and on a lee shore I'm going to put her if our stem holds out." Seizing the wheel and ringing "full ahead" he drove the Head for one of the schooners riding at anchor in the dark and struck her fair amidships, staving in her side and throwing her on her beam ends. She filled and sank, her mastheads going down first. All on board were drowned. "Ratsy" was overpowered again and put ashore at the Straits of Mackinac, and committed to an insane asylum for life. Several days after this disas-ter the swollen grain in the sunken schooner burst her hatches and poured out, and she floated to the surface. She was then identified as the Magellan, which had been carrying a crew of eight.

At four in the afternoon of December 4, 1904, a gale was run-ning from the east, on Lake Ontario, the Oliver Mowat passed Port Hope making for Bowmanville, with a load of coal from Oswego. The gale took the Mowat through the sleet until she hit a shoal half a mile from Oshawa. She was not seen due to snow squalls until next day. There was no lifeboat available at Toronto, Oshawa nor Port Hope, but a group of "harbour boys" at Port Hope got together and made up a volunteer crew, determined to do something. A fishboat was loaded into a wagon and taken to the railroad station. The Grand Trunk

Railway provided a shunting engine and a flat car. The boat was two miles east of the town. They rowed to the *Mowat* and managed to take off the crew of twelve men and a dog. Bailing steadily, they made it back to shore and got the men to Port Hope for medical attention, where the church bells were set ringing in thanksgiving. The *Mowat* was later hauled off the shoal and the "fishboat-lifeboat" was returned to Port Hope a week late. The bill sent to the government to cover cost of the use of the railway engine and flat car was $61. The government paid $40.

In the fall of 1872, a number of schooners were frozen in the St. Mary's River and forced to winter there. Among them were the *Ford* and the *Oak Leaf*. On Christmas Day the crew of the *Oak Leaf*, ten all told, left their vessel stripped for the winter, and began a march for Bay City, Michigan, through the wilderness. They carried provisions with them on a toboggan and made camp each night, cutting enough spruce boughs to shelter them from the bitter frost. They had firearms and supplemented their provisions with game. In two weeks they had reached Bay City, all in good health. The crew of the *Ford*, made a similar march to another destination. Sailors Encampment, at the Sault, may take its name from the fact that the sailors camped there before starting their long trek.

When the Drummond Island garrison was transferred to Penetanguishene in 1828, they were involved in the first recorded shipwreck of Georgian Bay. The schooner *Alice Hackett* was one of the vessels used to transfer the soldiers, stores and belongings of government people and settlers to the new station. Captain Hackett had already made one trip and this time, in addition to soldiers and supplies, he carried a man named Lepine with his wife and child, a tavern keeper named Frazer with thirteen barrels of whisky, along with considerable livestock and household furniture. No sooner had the little schooner got well underway from Drummond Island when Frazer opened shop. Before long, the captain and crew were in various stages of drunkenness. During the night, a storm blew up, but those in the vessel were in no condition to cope. They grounded on Fitzwilliam Island.

The crew and most of the passengers made it ashore. They lost much of the cargo, but, of course, they saved what was left of the whisky. Lepine's wife and infant were left on the wreck, forgotten in the drunken confusion. The woman fastened the baby to her back and tied herself to the mast where she remained throughout the storm. Next morning, the people on shore became sober enough to realize the woman and child were missing. They went out to the schooner in the yawl boat, which had been saved, and rescued them. The schooner was a total loss. Frazer and what was left of his barrels of whisky eventually reached Penetang where he established another tavern.

I have heard this period referred to many times as "the good old days."

CHAPTER 17

Fur Trade on the Lakes

THE FUR TRADERS HAD BEEN ACTIVE on the lakes for some fifty years before the first sail was ever seen. La Salle's little vessels on Lake Ontario in 1678 and the *Griffon* on the Upper Lakes in 1679 were built primarily with the fur trade in mind. The search for fur and the hope for wealth to be achieved through this trade brought many cases of untold hardship in the wilderness, injury and even frozen death among the first white trappers and traders.

The Natives reacted like covetous children when they saw the strange, glittery and amazing products of European industry. They were about to be extracted from the stone-age and catapulted into something entirely different. They had no idea of the real value of their furs, which they eagerly exchanged for worthless trinkets and trade goods, brass kettles, knives, guns, ornaments, brooches, beads, bits of glass, coats, blankets, calico, and, of course, gin, rum and whisky. The white traders, equally covetous but this time of wealth, took advantage of this gullibility.

Trapping took place all around each of the lakes, through the woods and prairies. The furs ranged from beaver, otter, muskrat, fisher, mink, fox to deer, but the "gold standard" of the industry was the beaver for which Europe had an insatiable demand, particularly for the beaver hats much in vogue at the time. At first the Natives would take their loads of furs to Montreal, Quebec and Trois Rivières to barter for the trinkets and trade goods. The early trade route from the Upper Lakes was along the north shore of Lake Huron and the French, Nipissing and Ottawa rivers to the St. Lawrence. But greed and an ever increasing need for fur drove the French further and further into the lake country.

The French-Canadian coureurs de bois readily adapted themselves to the wilderness. By 1680, when the total population of New France was only 10,000, some 800 men had entered the woods, mostly without licence, to trap and trade on their own account. Soon, large fleets of freight canoes, as many as 30 or even 60 at a time, always with a French Canadian on board, would appear each autumn, travelling along the north of Lake Huron, into Lake Michigan and Lake Superior. All winter the trappers would work in extremes of privation and hardship but would reappear in the late spring at the posts, their canoes bulging with fur and their bodies eager to carouse and celebrate.

Posts had been established early at Fort Frontenac, then Detroit, later at Mackinac, Sault Ste. Marie, Green Bay, Saginaw, Chicago, Grand Island, Grand Portage and many others. When Cadillac[1] founded Detroit in 1701, the Michigan Territories were one of the major fur producing areas. Detroit and Mackinac became the two most important trading centres. In the straits the post was moved, over the years, from St. Ignace to Michillimackinac on the south shore where the reconstructed fort now stands, to Mackinac Island.

In all the lake areas, to the mid-17th century, the French had been the predominant force. However, two French adventurers, Radisson and Grosseilliers,[2] who had spent time in the 1650s exploring Lake Superior, returning in the summer of 1660 with large cargos of furs, were instrumental in changing that. They tried to influence officials in New France and in France that the best source of beaver was north and west of Lake Superior, and further, that the best route to these riches was via Hudson Bay. They received no support, so took their story to England. The result was the founding of the Hudson's Bay Company in 1670, which, for many years, traded throughout this area and further west, in spite of French claims to the Lake Superior basin. However, in 1679, Du Lhut[3] reached the site of the present Duluth and claimed the surrounding land for France. In 1682, La Salle did the same for the Mississippi basin.

In 1687, the French, from Quebec, set out by canoe to attack the Hudson's Bay posts on James Bay and returned loaded with loot, principally beaver furs. On the pronouncement of war between France and Great Britain in 1689, the fur trade was curtailed for a while. The war from Europe moved into the lakes with the English from the American colonies, allied with the Iroquois First Nation, fighting against the French and their Native allies in French Canada. There were repeated bloody battles and loss of life on both sides. In 1690, Quebec was attacked by a fleet of thirty ships from Boston, under the leadership of Sir William Phipps, Governor of Massachusetts. The attack failed. All of these escapades and attacks interfered with the fur trade. One year there would be a shortfall, and the next year such a surplus of beaver that as they tried to unload the looted pelts in Paris, the government had to suspend the fur trade temporarily.

By 1693, the fur trade was re-established. However, the English now had a good foothold via Hudson Bay, and were extending their influence beyond the Upper Lakes and the northwest into the American West. In 1713, under the terms of the Treaty of Utrecht, France yielded the commerce of Hudson's Bay to the English, but they still attempted to control and build up trade around Lake Superior and further west. Great adventures were undertaken but all this ended for France soon after the defeat by the British at Quebec in 1759. French authority left the lakes forever, but the French coureurs de bois merely changed allegiance to the new British masters, and carried on.

The Hudson's Bay Company generally worked far north of the lakes and further west. The Canadian-based North West Company was constituted to trade on the lakes and streams draining into the lakes from the north and west.[4] The newer company had been organized in 1783 and had some 2,000 men, factors, clerks, interpreters, traders

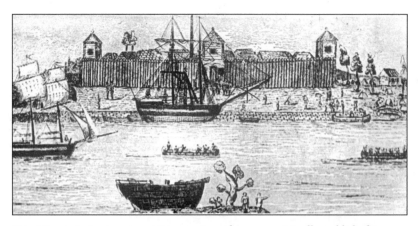

Fort Kaministiquia, *circa 1805, artist unknown, originally published in*
Father Aeneas McDonell Dawson's Our Strength and their Strength
(Ottawa, 1870). Sieur du Lhut built the first Fort Kaministiquia around
1683 and in 1803 the North West Company held its first "rendezvous"
there. Note the schooners, batteaux and canoes at the wharf, voyageur tents
to the left of newly erected palisades and the Native component to the right.
Courtesy of Library and Archives, C-24733.

and trappers, working for it. Their furs were brought down to
Montreal and shipped to London. American merchants could only
buy them via London. Another Canadian company was the smaller
Mackinac Company, which traded below or south of the lakes. Its
largest post was at Mackinac Island. The company was reaping half a
million dollars worth of fur every year from the Wisconsin Territory
and the upper Mississippi and Missouri basins.

This situation was about to be changed and the man who was
going to do it was John Jacob Astor. A poor immigrant boy, born on
July 17, 1763, at Waldorf, Germany, he arrived in America in January
1784, and started out as a delivery boy for his brother who ran a
bakery in New York City. He soon found a job with a furrier, and, in
a small way, was buying and selling furs in his own name soon after.
Before long he was shipping furs to England and importing musical
instruments into New York: flutes, clarinets, fifes, chamber organs
and sheet music. He was making a good profit in both directions. By
1790, he was dealing in futures on the market in Montreal, and by

1800, he was selling furs in Canton, China, and bringing back tea and brocade to sell in America. The famous Hotel Waldorf Astoria in New York City is named in his honour. In April 1808, he established the American Fur Company and three years later Fort Astoria was established on the Pacific coast.

Although the fur trade continued to make Astor extremely wealthy for many years, it reached its peak in the early 1830s. Astor, an expert in timing, sold out in 1834 and while the empire did not disappear for many years, the fur trade was on the decline. The company shifted its interests into the timber and land speculation business. The tide of immigrants provided a good market and the company continued to prosper from their need for land and homes.

While the story of this period makes very fascinating reading, the focus is to be on sail in the Great Lakes. The only sailing craft in this early era were La Salle's ships and the few built at Black Rock and Detroit in the late 18th century. These craft, and the ones that followed in the trade up to the war, were described earlier. As trade moved from the Nipissing-Ottawa route to the Great Lakes, these small ships were kept very busy.

In the increasing trade after the war, the smaller ships would carry flour, clothing, liquor, trade goods to the posts in the northwest and to the settlers' communities. They would return loaded with peltry. As early as 1793, it is reported that 4,000 bushels of Indian corn and 200,000 pounds of flour were shipped from Detroit to Mackinac Island and Sault Ste. Marie. This trade continued until the settlers could support themselves and even produce crops that they could trade with others. In 1834, Astor's American Fur Company felt the need of a large vessel for the Upper Lakes business. Ramsay Crooks, who had been Astor's agent for many years, was in charge, and a vessel of 112 tons was built.

The frame timbers and planks of white oak were cut at Black River, Ohio, during the winter and in April 1835 they were shipped on board the schooner *Bridget* to the Sault. The materials were then hauled over the portage and the keel for the new vessel was laid on the shores of Lake Superior on the 17th of May. This first vessel to be built and launched by Americans on Lake Superior, was given the name *John Jacob Astor*. It sailed on the 15th of August, and on the 26th of the same month, Captain Charles C. Stanard regrettably discovered the famous rock which now bears his name. A lighthouse was later built there and named Stanard's Rock Light. The *Astor* sailed Lake Superior for nearly fifty years. It was wrecked as it lay at anchor in Copper Harbor on Sept. 21, 1884. A violent storm caused the cable to part and she was driven onto the rocky shore.

The American Fur Company built another vessel, the *Madaline* in 1837, and, in 1838, the schooner *William Webster* (73 tons) was added to the fleet. The latter was sent down the St. Mary's Rapids in 1842 to join the more profitable trade on lakes Huron and Michigan. In 1836, the Company built, the 100-foot long brigantine, *Ramsay Crooks*, at Detroit. She was a handsome vessel of 247 tons that carried supplies to Mackinac and the Sault for ten years, bringing back load after load of furs and other products to Detroit. She was the last vessel built for the fur trade on the Great Lakes.

The virtual monopoly of the British Hudson's Bay Company and the Canadian North West Company had been a major deterrent to Astor's ambitions, and, when Jay's Treaty of 1796[5] was signed, he felt he could expand at top speed into the western fur trade. When Britain gave up Mackinac and Detroit to the Americans, Astor established bases at both places. By 1808 he had the trade well in hand and had changed his company name to the American Fur Company, of which he was the sole owner. His place in the War of 1812 has been recounted earlier.

Astor still had rivals, one of which was the government itself, and he set out to win a monopoly. Some traders plied the Natives with liquor unscrupulously. A few cents worth of whisky won the traders three or four dollars worth of furs. The American Fur Company had fewer scruples than its rivals. Colonel Josiah Snelling, commander of the American military post at Detroit, reported that 3,300 gallons of whisky and 2,500 gallons of high wines had been shipped to the American Fur Company at Mackinac in 1825 from Detroit alone. The high wines were nearly pure alcohol, diluted to make "firewater." Of course, all fur trading companies on both sides of the border were guilty of the same unprincipled behaviour with the Native Peoples.

The American government set up its own trading posts to deal directly with the Aboriginals in an attempt to reduce the effects of the dishonest and unscrupulous traders. Thus, it created competition with Astor who did not like this situation. He went to Washington in 1816, where he still had great influence, and was instrumental in lobbying for a new law that refused trading licences to all but American citizens. This action was aimed at the British at Fond du Lac and other western posts. Then he induced the government to establish military posts to protect his own men and to enforce the new law. When the "foreigners" (those traders from Canada) were driven out, he persuaded the government to abolish its own trading posts and Astor took them over. He was a master of manipulation to achieve his own purposes.

Next, through his monopolistic practices, and the utilization of his vast financial resources, he was able to force many of his competitors out of business or buy them up at distress prices. He was exceptionally ruthless in dealing with competitors. He would send his traders into their territory with orders to buy at any price. Then, in the selling markets of the seaboard, he would sell at discount prices. He could absorb the losses but his competitors could not and many went into bankruptcy. He bought out the Canadian Mackinaw (Michilmackinac) Company and absorbed it into the American Fur Company.

Immediately after the War of 1812, Astor established his headquarters on Mackinac Island. From here, he virtually controlled the entire industry in America, and part of it in Canada. He preferred to employ the French-Canadian voyageurs who seemed much more compliant and willing to do his bidding than the American trappers. His agent, Ramsay Crooks, wrote that the Americans "…were too independent to submit quietly to proper control," but the Canadians had "…that temper of mind to render him patient, docile and persevering, in short they are a people harmless in themselves whose habits of submission fit them peculiarly for our business."

CHAPTER 18

Fishing on the Lakes

FOR THOSE WHO HAVE GONE SPORT FISHING on the lakes in recent years, stories of multitudes of pickerel, of tons of salmon, of hundreds of barrels of herring and whitefish and similar stories are apt to be taken as just so much overstatement and extreme exaggeration. If, like the writer, you have tried for hours to hook a big one and have eventually given up in disgust, you will have trouble believing that catches in the olden days were frequently so great that the fishermen were at a loss as to how to dispose of them profitably. You will feel more than disgust at the practices, which, in their greed and ignorance, destroyed this wonderful resource.

Fish had been a staple of the Natives' diet for countless centuries before the Europeans appeared an the scene. Fish and corn were the main items of their menu, which many early writers described as monotonous. These same huge quantities of fish continued in the lakes until the early 1800s, in fact, in some areas until the end of the century. As early as 1670, Radisson reported on the Native fisheries at Sault Ste Marie. John Johnston in his *Account of Lake Superior 1792-1807*, described the Natives of Grand Island going fishing every calm night with "flambeaux,"[1] and noted, "They take as

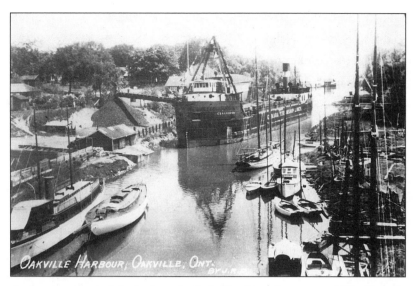

A photo postcard of the harbour in Oakville, Ontario, c. 1940. The Canada Steamship Lines' steamship, the Coalhaven, *can be seen unloading coal on the east bank of the Sixteen Mile Creek. A large steam yacht is in the left foreground, two masts of a larger sailing vessel are visible in the right fore-ground and a variety of smaller sailboats are along the right side of the harbour. Today, Oakville can boast of a large collection of pleasure yachts in modern marina settings, a great change from the earlier days of commercial maritime activity and shipbuilding.* Courtesy of Walter Lewis, Maritime History of the Great Lakes webmaster.

fine trout and whitefish as are found in any part of the lakes." He mentions one taken off the north of Montreal Island as weighing fifty-two pounds. Other early writers talk of filling canoes to the gun-wales with fish in a very short period of time.

Nor were the best fisheries always to be found in Lake Superior. Writing about life on the north shore of Lake Ontario, of Oakville and the Sixteen Mile Creek in particular during the early 1800s, Hazel Mathews says, "In the Spring the Sixteen abounded with Atlantic Salmon; in fact, one eighteenth-century French map shows it as 'Rivière au Saumon.' The fish swam up the St. Lawrence into Lake Ontario in great numbers to spawn in rivers and creeks where they were taken in great quantities. Weighing from fifteen to eight-een pounds, the salmon were easily caught, a night's catch sometimes filling eight or ten barrels. When salted down the 200 pound barrels sold for 30s or 35s each."[2]

She also quotes a Mr. Warr who described fishing the Sixteen thus, "The mode of fishing practiced by the Indians is exceedingly interesting. The operation is carried on at night; two men generally steal along with the utmost caution in their canoe; the one uses the paddle, the other the spear; the former sits in the stern, the latter stands in the bow of the boat; they invariably carry a large piece of pine lighting in a grate which is so arranged as to cast a strong glare upon the water and enable the fisherman to see the fish, which he strikes with his harpoon with unerring aim, and instantly throws it into the boat. In this way they continue night after night…It need scarcely be observed that it requires both the eye and the aim of the Indian to be a successful angler after this manner; and yet the author has met with gentlemen who were not only quite captivated with but generally successful in these nocturnal sports of the native tribes.[3]" She goes on the describe William Howes who lived about nine miles up the creek as stating that he had seen "…wagon loads of beautiful salmon taken out there. They were speared with pitchforks." Although Mrs. Mathews writes of the Sixteen Mile Creek only, there is no reason to believe that other streams and rivers flowing into Lake Ontario were not similarly blessed.

The whitefish of Lake Superior and Lake Huron were famous from early days. Mrs. Anna Jameson who toured this area by canoe in the mid-1830s wrote, "Here, at the foot of the rapids, the celebrated whitefish of the lakes is caught. The people down below [on the shores of the Lower Lakes] who boast of the excellence of the whitefish, really know nothing of the matter. There is no more comparison between the whitefish of the lower lakes and the whitefish of St. Mary's, than between the plaice and the turbot, or between a clam and a Sandwich oyster. I ought to be a judge, who having eaten them fresh out of the river four times a day, and I declare to you that I have never tasted anything of the fish kind half so exquisite. It is said by Alexander Henry that people never tire of them. Mr. McMurray, missionary at the Canadian Sault, tells me that he has eaten them every day of his life for seven years."[4]

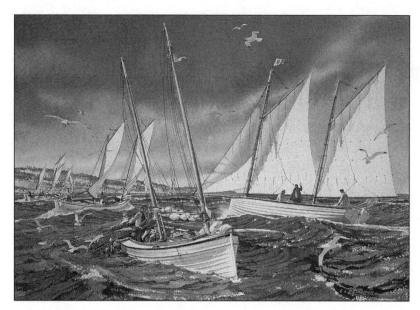

Fishing from small sailboats was a common means of livelihood out on the lakes in the mid-1800s to the close of the nineteenth century. Featured in the centre is a Collingwood skiff. Behind her to the left is a Mackinaw and to the right is a Huron boat. Far over to the left is a three-masted Huron boat, the Belle Jean Ann *of Goderich.* Charles L. Peterson, artist.

Mrs. Jameson was ecstatic over the skills of these Native fishermen. Drawing on her observations from touring in Italy, she declared, "I used to admire the fishermen on the Arno and those on the Laguna and above all the Neapolitan fishermen hauling in their nets, or diving like ducks, but I never saw anything like these Indians. The manner in which they keep their position upon a footing of a few inches, is to me as incomprehensible as the beauty of their forms and attitudes, swayed by every movement and turn of their dancing, fragile barks, is admirable."[5]

The Natives would either dry the fish over racks in the sun, thus preserving them for a time, or else they would be frozen and kept all winter. With the coming of the white man, the need for larger quantities of fish increased, along with it the need for faster ways of catching them. Netting was introduced early in the 19th century, and the nets were handled from boats, sometimes rowboats, but soon small sailboats were used.

By the time the first maps were made, the islands of the Saugeen shore were known for the fish that congregated in their vicinity. The name, Fishing Islands, appears on the Bayfield maps of 1820, but the first record of commercial fishing describes events in 1831, when Alexander McGregor of Goderich explored this coast and found an abundance of the kinds of fish that were in commercial demand: herring, whitefish and lake trout. One spot was favoured above all others by herring and whitefish. Here, in their seasons, these two species came together in schools so dense that the fish, like Pacific salmon crowding upstream to their spawning beds, fairly lifted each other out of the water. The shoals, the rocky banks and the networks of pools and winding channels among the Fishing Islands were their favourite spots.

McGregor bought a stock of seines, along with twine and kit for repairing them, and drying racks, to be added to his fleet of two-masted schooners and rowboats. He loaded aboard many barrels and a quantity of rock salt. The fish were practically begging to be caught, but McGregor had neglected to figure out what he was going to do with them. Not until 1834 did McGregor find the market he needed, when, in that year, he made a contract with a Detroit company to deliver 3,000 barrels of salted whitefish and herring. The price was $1 per barrel, the company to assume the cost of cleaning and packing all fish delivered. The business thrived, and proof of the story comes from the writings of a famous missionary to the Natives, the Reverend James Evans who spent a day at the Saugeen Fishing Islands preaching to the fishermen of the Huron Fishing Company. He wrote, "This is a fine fishery, sometimes four hundred barrels of herring are caught at one single haul of the seine."[6] There is one report of a catch of 350 tons, half of which had to be let go because McGregor did not have sufficient salt to preserve them.

McGregor had other troubles. In the autumn of 1835, one of his ships ran aground thirty-six miles north of Goderich and was frozen in for the entire winter. This did not stop him. He decided to deliver the cargo by sleigh, since he could not do it by water. In his diary, the Laird of Goderich, William "Tiger" Dunlop, states that on January 29, 1836, and again on March 18, he saw McGregor pass through

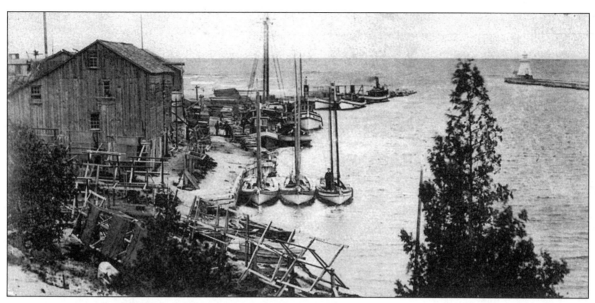

This postcard of the mouth of the Saugeen River was mailed in 1907. It is likely that the image was taken just before the end of the nineteenth century as it shows the other range light. While the fleet is remarkably similar to that shown in the pre-1883 photo of the area, there have been many more buildings constructed. Courtesy of Paul Carroll.

Goderich on his way to the imprisoned schooner for a load of salted fish, each time driving a train of four sledges.

The method of fishing is most interesting, as documented for us by Norman Robertson in his book, *History of the County of Bruce*, published in 1906. It was Captain McGregor's practice to post a man in a tall tree to enable him to get a clear view of the expanse frequented by the schooling fish. There the watcher stayed patiently, sometimes for many tedious hours, looking much like a kingfisher on a branch overhanging a pool. What he sought was a first glint of a sheet of sparkling silver moving swiftly over the water. The instant he spied it, he shouted his discovery to the men on the ground. Without delay, they launched their large, heavy rowboats, which, with sterns piled high with the long seine nets, were held ready for the spotter's call. Guided by his signals, they steered straight for the school of fish, dropped their nets and began drawing them in a great curve that would encircle the swarming mass. The circle completed, the animated

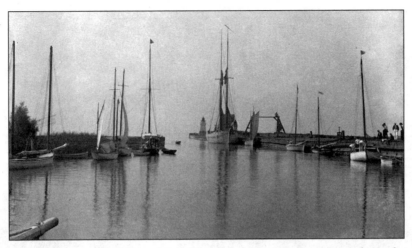

Even as the age of sail began its decline and the era of steam-powered vessels became well entrenched in maritime transportation, the presence of sailing vessels in Port Dover was still predominate in the first decade of the 1900s. Witness this photograph showing the Eliza Allen *and a number of small sloops, a sailing skiff and various fishing boats, circa 1905.* Courtesy of the Port Dover Harbour Museum.

"kettle of fish" was laboriously dragged shoreward.[7] The business prospered and Captain McGregor built facilities to house his men on Main Station Island, offshore from Oliphant (north of Southampton) in the Fishing Islands. The large stone building was the first structure to be erected for many miles around and the rough remains were still visible not many years ago.

Commercial fishing started even earlier on Lake Erie, in the Detroit River, the Maumee River and around the Pass Islands. Every possible source of food was made use of by the armies of both countries during the War of 1812. Seine nets were used from the beginning, and by 1826 Detroit was shipping whitefish and lake trout, both salted and barrelled, to the eastern markets. The catch included, in addition, herring, yellow pike, perch and the bass that gave the islands of Lake Erie their name. Boats went out from Sandusky, Port Stanley, Erie, Port Dover and just about every other port on both sides of the lake.

While some commercial fishing was done with hook and line, and some was done through the ice in winter, this does not concern our subject. The majority of fishing was with nets of one sort or another. Gill nets were used from a very early date. It is said that the first nets were made from linen ravelled from clothing by the fishermen's wives. The nets were made by hand and were secured on the bottom where they stood upright in the manner of a tennis net. The principle was that the fish would not see them and would swim headlong into the meshes and be caught behind the head or by the gill covers. The nets were set from little fishing boats that got out to the fishing grounds by "ash breeze" if near shore, or under sail if further out. The term refers to a sequence that would have a small boat tied ahead of the main ship, becalmed, to row forward, towing the larger vessel, to reach a new patch of wind.

The nets were stored neatly in boxes and were buoyed up by wooden floats at the top and held down by stones at the bottom. Later this evolved into cast-lead sinkers and cedar floats. One still sees these floats, in plastic, on the lakes, marked by flags or sometimes by the ubiquitous Javex bottle. The nets were raised and lowered over the stern or quarter of the small work boats of the fishermen, with usually two or three men assigned to each boat.

Trout were taken on long "trot" lines to which were attached 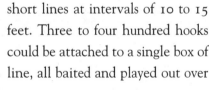 short lines at intervals of 10 to 15 feet. Three to four hundred hooks could be attached to a single box of line, all baited and played out over

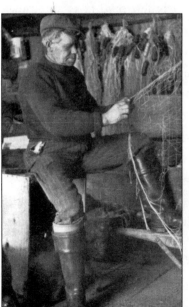

While temporary repairs to fish nets were made onboard, or as nets were trailed on to drying reels, the major repairs were made during the long winter months. Sailors sat in dark shanties, heated by pot-bellied stoves, and laboured long hours. They would often gam about the seasons gone by – there were endless tales to tell. In this photo, L.H. (Louie) Macleod, a well-known Bayfield fisherman, mends his nets in a shanty alongside the Bayfield River. Courtesy of Phil Gemeinhardt.

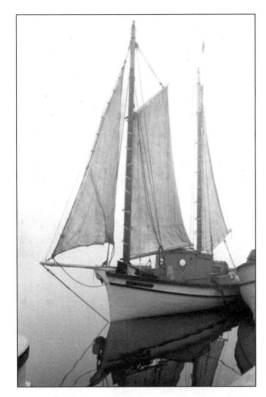

The serenity of Lake Huron is notable in this image (c. 1940) of the fishing vessel, Helen Macleod II *at Bayfield. She is becalmed, drying her sails while rafted to a sister ship at dockside. She is reputed to be the last working Huron boat on the lakes.* Courtesy of the Bayfield Archives.

the stern as the boat moved along slowly. The line would lie at the bottom of the lake, stretched out for many miles. Each line was raised periodically and a newly baited line lowered in its place.

Pound nets that, instead of meshing the fish led them through a passage or tunnel into the "pot," were introduced in the mid-1800s, and soon replaced other types in some areas. Trap nets and fyke nets (a long bag net distended by hoops), are variations of the pound nets. They are all set at depths of up to 90 feet.

It is the type of boats used by the fishermen that is more of our concern here, for the vessels that carried the processed catch to market, either to the east or to the settlements at the more remote parts of the lakes, have already been discussed. Considering that small sail craft were used in all the Great Lakes and that they were in use for something around 100 years, surprisingly few hard facts are known about them.

In general, these small craft were built in so many places and boat yards, that the pedigree of many of the types is extremely obscure. Only a few have been identified as distinct types and there is much about them that is still disputed today. While the serious student will be concerned with even minor differences, the needs in all the lakes were similar and the appearance of the majority of the types, to the non-scholar, showed many features in common.

All were in the size range from 18 to 40 feet long, and by far the majority were between 32 and 38 feet. Almost all had centreboards of one form or another. A few had only one mast and one boat of record had three, but the majority were two-masted.

Countless carpenters would have built their own boats after seeing one that appealed to them, then gone into the business. Some

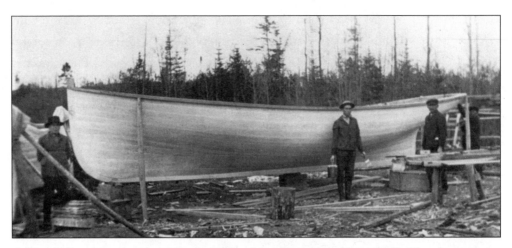

A large hull nearing completion at the Harbor Island boatyard of Jesse Wells Church, c. 1905. It was fitted with an inboard engine for fishing. J.W. Church came on the scene relatively late, and as he kept a journal from 1845 to 1910, much is known of his boat-building activities. Harbor Island is near the mouth of the St. Mary's River where it empties into Lake Huron. Courtesy of Roger Swanson.

experienced builders came to the lakes bringing their knowledge from the seaboard or from Europe. We know little about these builders. Most did not leave their names on the records, or, if they did, the record has not come to light. A few names have surfaced and fewer models yet can be attributed to these builders with any degree of certainty. Some names have been given credit though they perhaps duplicated or modified one of the already known types.

In 1848, two Scotsmen purchased the Huron Fishing Company from McGregor. Captain John Spence and Captain William F. Kennedy had been ship's carpenters for the Hudson's Bay Company. Spence was born in Birsby, in the Orkneys, in 1815, and served his apprenticeship in the shipyards of Stromness where Arctic whalers fitted out and local boats were built. The two pioneers would have known what type of vessel they felt was best-suited to their chosen trade, and they would know how to build it. The Huron boat certainly resembles the large clinker-built herring boats of North Britain, which had two masts and lugsails, as did the early Huron boats built at Goderich and other ports on Lake Huron.

Many of the fine schooners sailing out of Goderich were built right in the local harbour. Soon after his arrival in this new town, John Galt initiated the building of a Canada Company boat.[8] But it was not until after a second start that this first commercial vessel, a steam-powered sidewheeler, the *Minnesetung* was finally launched in 1832.

John Thornton and George Ault continued building a variety of boats during these early years. These included different types of sailing vessels and sail yachts, according to Captain Robert A. Sinclair, as chronicled in his *Winds Over Lake Huron*, published in the 1960s. Then Henry Marlton and his son William, who had first built sailing vessels on the harbour flats, established a yard on Ship Island, a large alluvial island in the northeast corner of Goderich's commercial harbour basin. According to Captain Sinclair, "Mr. Marlton was credited with a remarkable memory, and if he went on board one of the ships

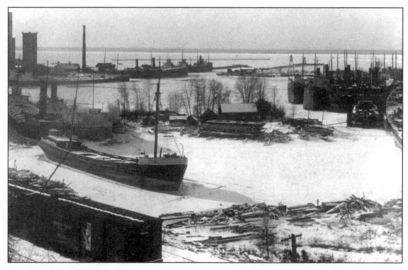

As the era of sail came to a close, grand vessels became derelicts, often abandoned at the back of a harbour, eventually to be towed away to a nearby shallow water grave and scuttled. Shipbuilding facilities, which could not be switched to keep pace with the new age of steam-powered craft, tried to sustain activity by building work dredges and scows. Such was the fate of the famed Marlton Shipyards on Ship Island (Goderich), the birthplace of dozens of magnificent sailing vessels, shown here in her final years. A scow in the slipways is ready for launching next spring, photo c. 1920. Courtesy of the Huron County Museum.

to obtain some measurements and then was accosted by someone on his way down about an entirely different matter, he was still able to keep the figures in his head. At one time some of his workmen were about to smooth out some frames when he stopped them saying that such a beautiful job of adze work should be left for all to see and admire."[9]

In the period 1849 to 1907, the Marltons built nearly seventy schooners, tugs and steamers. These included the schooners *Annexation*, the *Stanley*, the *Shade*, the *N. Scott*, the *Tecumseh*, the *Jennie Rumball*, the *Nemesis*, the yacht *Alarm* and the *Greyhound*. They ran from 20 to 210 gross tons and were up to 111 feet in length.

One of the most famous Marlton ships was the schooner *Sephie*, built in 1889 for Joseph Williams and used in the lumber trade. She ultimately was sold across the Atlantic in 1917, and remained in service there after the First World War. Among their major achievements, according to Mac Campbell of Goderich, were the two vessels, the *Caribou* and the *Manitou*, both passenger ships about 200 feet in length. The *Caribou* ran a ferry for passengers and freight between Tobermory and South Baymouth, and other ports in the Manitoulin Island-North Channel area.

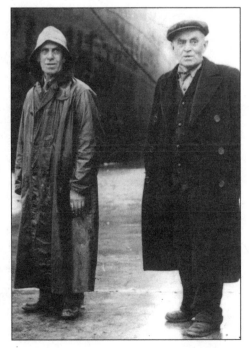

Captain Bert MacDonald (left) and his brother Reddy, sons of Captain John MacDonald, c. 1940s. Reddy was a fisherman who sailed in any weather and survived many storms. His navigation abilities and his courage were always augmented with strong spirits of the liquid kind. Captain Bert was a boat builder and a tug captain. His life-saving accomplishments were legendary over many decades. In his later life he spent hours teaching youngsters to swim in the deep waters between the Goderich piers, while they were tethered to a safety line. Bert ran the wooden tugs, the Captain John *and the* Annamac, *the last of their kind to be used at Goderich Harbour. He also introduced the* Donald Bert, *the first of three steel-hulled work tugs that are still in use in Goderich Harbour today.* Courtesy of the Huron County Museum.

Shipbuilding at Goderich has really never ceased. Following the Marltons, Bill "Spike" Bermingham was a business partner of "Big" Bill Forrest, the builder of dredges, barges and other work vessels, and who occupied Ship Island in Goderich Harbour. Bill ran the finance and office matters; Forrest was the hands-on "grunt" man. Together they constructed the first portions of the Goderich Harbour break-walls in the early 1900s, after several failed attempts by other contractors whose work was washed out by fierce storms.[10]

In the second decade of this century, Bert MacDonald, a renowned waterman built wooden fishing tugs for his brothers Mac and Reddy, and other small sailing craft. In the post war years of the Second World War, George Mathieson operated a thriving industry building steel tugs. Later in the 1960s Bruce MacDonald utilized modern materials and produced fibreglass sailing dinghies and built at least one fine schooner, the *Wanderer*. In the 1970s and 80s, Bob Patterson, in his then-modern Huronic Metal Industries factory, built a steel sailing craft, the *Goderich 35*. Today, H. Ted Gozzard and family build several variations of sailing vessels from 31 to 47 feet in length, in sloop, cutter and ketch-rigged configurations and custom power and sail to 70 feet. His company is the last surviving Canadian builder of luxury sailing yachts of size.[11]

The early days of sail and the colourful schooners saw such famous Goderich sailors as Captains Andrew and John Bogie, Captain Thomas Dancey and the well-known Captain John MacDonald. The lake boats have always attracted the young townsmen and many have taken to the lake and its boats for their livelihood. From the days of Captain John, the name MacDonald, often spelled Macdonald, was to become a widely known Goderich sailing name. It is reported that Mr. Bermingham once made the remark, "If one were to yell 'MacDonald' at the harbour, he would be run down in the stampede."

Huron boats, 24 to 40 feet long, became very common on the Upper Lakes. They made excellent craft for the fishermen, and were also used as small cargo vessels. They were very seaworthy and sufficiently shallow draft to get into many coves and river mouths for protection whenever necessary.

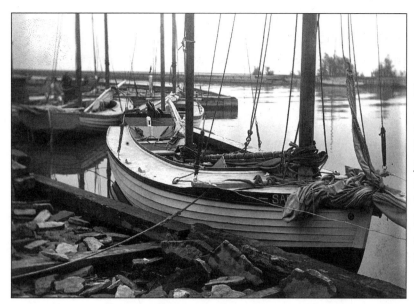

Bronte Harbour, 1910, showing several Huron boats, as used for pleasure. Courtesy of Walter Lewis, Maritime History of the Great Lakes webmaster.

It seems today that any boat that was built, or even sailed in the vicinity of Mackinaw, the Straits or the Island of Mackinac took the name "Mackinaw boat." It is hard to prove that any specific type either originated, or was, in fact, extensively built there.

From the early days of the European explorer, trader or settler, stories have come down to us about Mackinaw boats. Many appear to have referred to the French-Canadian bateaux, however, there does not appear to be any connection between the bateaux and the sail craft which followed. There are three principal categories of craft (and variations of each) that are most commonly referred to as Mackinaw boats.

The Collingwood skiff was a double-ender some 26 to 36 feet long, with a straight stem and a marked rake to the stern post on which was hung an outboard rudder. They were either lapstrake or carvel built and were originally fitted with boiler-plate centreboards, but this was changed in later years to heavy wooden boards. Early photographs, probably taken in the 1800s, show single-masted as well as two-masted versions, and lugsails as well as gaff sails. As the style evolved, the most common rig included a jib attached to a long bowsprit, severely hogged down. Many hundreds of these were built in the 19th century and were used on all the lakes. They served not only for fishing but as the family "flivver." In the early to mid-1800s, these skiffs began to be built for yachting. At one time there were twenty or thirty in the Toronto area used for pleasure and one, at least, has survived into the 1970s, on which I had the pleasure of sailing. It was authentic, except for the fact that she carried dacron sails in lieu of cotton. She was built at Collingwood around 1923.

The Huron boat was not dissimilar but had a wide transom and therefore a much greater cargo carrying capacity. Some evolved with clipper bows, referred to as "chicken beak" and one at least, the *Belle Jean Anne* of Goderich, had three masts, The Huron boat is very much like a small version of the larger lake schooners. The *Helen MacLeod II*, whose hull is resting in a shed near Bayfield, is reputed to be the last working fishing vessel of this type on the lakes. Another version was quite similar to the Collingwood skiff with a fine counter stern. No record has appeared as to who first built it or when.

Around the year 1854, a boat builder named William Watts immigrated from Ireland and started building boats on one of the Toronto Islands. They were 20 feet long, double-ended, clinker-built with sprit sails, sloop- or ketch- rigged. In 1858, Watts moved to Collingwood and continued to build his skiffs for the local fishermen.

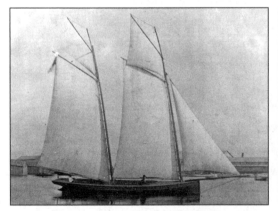 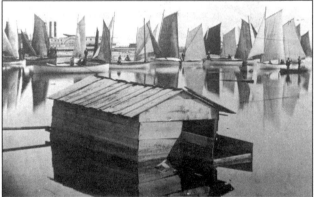

Left: The Mocking Bird, *a Mackinaw boat, was built as a pleasure yacht by William Watts of Collingwood, photo c. 1970s. Right: A view of a fishing fleet of Collingwood skiffs celebrating the 24th of May in the late 1880s.* Courtesy of the Collingwood Museum.

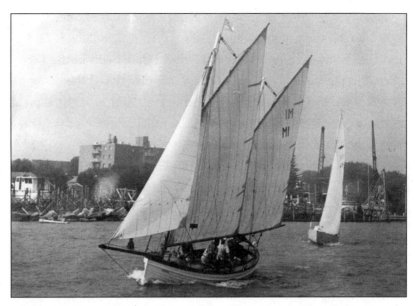

I first met Ken Jones and his Nahama in 1982. He had already owned her for 30 years and was quite an expert on the history of the early fishing boats. The Nahama was built in Collingwood in 1923 by Nathaniel Watts. She is 26' 3 1/2" on deck with a 12-foot bowsprit. Her working sail was 465 square feet. Experts disagree on the details and lineage of the Collingwood skiff and the Huron boat. Still, they are something to enjoy! She was probably the last of her type to sail on Lake Ontario, perhaps on all of the Great Lakes.

In all probability someone else on Lake Ontario moved in to fill the gap in the Toronto market, left by William Watts' withdrawal from the area. The same type of skiff appears in old photos from as far away as Sacket's Harbor at the eastern end of Lake Ontario. In any event, Watts' business prospered in Collingwood, building his boats and selling them all around the lakes on both sides of the border. Over time the models became larger in order to permit the fishermen to go farther afield.

The sprit sail gave way to the gaff rig, a long bowsprit and jib were added, but the masts were otherwise unstayed. The size increased to 35 feet on deck and a few were fitted with half-deck and a small cuddy cabin. The Watts family continued to build skiffs into the 1900s and built the yacht *Nahama*, on which I enjoyed a sail. They built other types as well, particularly the Huron boat in both carvel as well as lapstrake versions. No record is available as to numbers but it probably was up in the hundreds. There are records of some fishing companies on the Canadian shores of Lake Huron and Georgian Bay having as many as thirty-five of the skiffs in their fleets in the 1880s. There is no irrefutable proof that the Watts introduced the design to the lakes for, in short order, it was being built and used throughout all the lakes and may well have been the most common of the three recognized versions of the Mackinaw boat.

It is interesting to note the striking similarity between the rig as it finally evolved on the lakes and that of the Brocklebank shallop as built at Whitehaven in England in 1806. Could this have been coincidence or natural evolvement, or was the information that led to the construction of similar vessels here brought out to the lakes by an early immigrant?

Where did the sail plan originate? Was it natural evolution? This sketch shows the builder's plan of a shallop, built in 1806 by Brocklebank at Whitehaven, England. Taken from Sailing Ships *1775–1815* and reproduced, with permission, by David MacGregor.

CHAPTER 19

The Timber Droghers

IT IS DIFFICULT FOR US TODAY TO IMAGINE the vast timber wealth that covered the Great Lakes basin two hundred years ago. Apart from a few rocky outcroppings, scattered savannas and patches of sand dunes, it was entirely covered with vast stands of pine, oak, maple, walnut, beech, elm, hemlock and other trees.

Greedy harvesting of the timber and wanton destruction of anything less than the best, coupled with careless or deliberate burning, have almost totally destroyed this immense resource, leaving little or nothing for our children. The removal of timber started first in the St. Lawrence and Ottawa valleys. From the shores of Lake Ontario, from east and south, timbers were shipped out in the 1700s for building ships in England, for sale in the seaboard markets. A relatively small proportion was used for local building.

Thousands upon thousands of trees were felled for local ship-building during the War of 1812 and for ships of commerce in the following years. But this was a mere pittance compared with the growth of the timber harvesting and devastation to follow through the mid-1800s and to reach a peak around 1890.

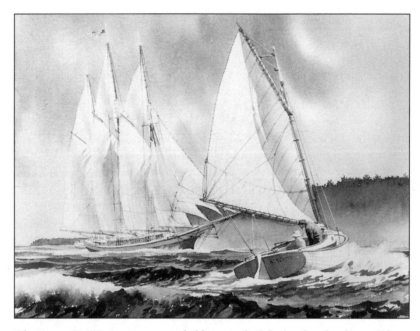

The Annie M Peterson *was probably typical of the lumber droghers of the late 1800s. Built at Green Bay, Wisconsin, in 1884, she was registered at 1200 tons and for many years was regarded locally as the fastest ship on the lakes.* Charles L. Peterson, artist.

It is possible to look at one area alone, the State of Michigan, as what happened there is not really any different from what took place in other areas bordering the lakes. Lumber was shipped out of every harbour where a ship could put in, and on every shape and size of craft available. Every river large enough to create a safe harbour and with sufficient flow to transport the logs cut in the winter became a major timber port with from one to many sawmills on its banks.

The winding Saginaw River, flowing through Bay City into Saginaw Bay, was typical. At the peak of the industry, as one writer has said, sixty mills along the Saginaw cut over a billion feet of lumber annually, and over a thousand lumber droghers,[1] a sailing boat especially designed and built for hauling lumber, per month loaded up along its shores with the finest clear white pine in the world. Trees five to six feet in diameter at the bole were not uncommon. The first steam mill on the river was built in the 1830s and the engine used was claimed to be salvaged from the steamship *Superior*, which, in turn, got it from the ill-fated *Walk-In-The-Water* built in 1818. The sawmill was in operation until 1854, when it was destroyed by fire.

Some of the timber cut here was used in shipyards interspaced between the sawmills, for building the ships that would carry away the wealth of the land. Thurlow Weed, writing in the *Albany Evening Journal* in 1847 of a trip by steamer from Buffalo to Chicago and back, mentions the vast consumption of wood on the trip:

> At 8.30 on July 2nd we came alongside a dock on the Canadian shore [in the St. Clair River], to take on wood. An hundred and six cords of wood, hickory, maple, beech and oak were seized by the deck-hands, steerage passengers, etc., and soon transferred from the dock to the boat… I learn that the *Empire* on a single trip consumes over 600 cords of wood. This requires for each trip the clearing up of over ten acres of well-wooded land.

At that time there were over 3,000 boats on the Erie Canal alone, most of which would be steam-powered. On the lakes there were 150 steamships, both sidewheelers and propellers. It is no wonder that the timber stands along the shores disappeared so rapidly.

The rampant harvesting of Michigan forests continued until around 1885, then started to decline. Some five hundred ships of all descriptions were in use at the time and around 8,000 cargos of timber would be carried in one season. Over 8,000 lumberjacks worked in the industry around the lakes. As the trees within the economical hauling distance of the Saginaw and its tributaries were all cut down, the mills were dismantled and moved to other rivers in the state, and finally to even more remote forests. When the best of southern Michigan had been harvested, they moved to Superior, to Georgian Bay and the Bruce Peninsula.

In *Georgian Bay, the Sixth Great Lake*, James Barry tells of the case of one Michigan lumberman from Saginaw who was having trouble

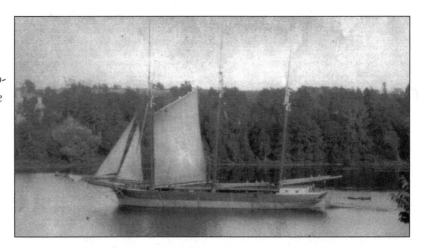

This timber drogher, the Queen of the Lakes, *was photographed in the Bay of Quinte. She was lost in 1906.* Courtesy of the Archives and Collection Society, Picton. Ontario.

with his creditors and took drastic action to outwit them. One night he left a bottle of whisky where the creditors' watchman would find it and a short time later, two tugs and two lighters pulled up to the mill, where the machinery had already been dismantled and was locked up. The machinery and everything else, even the siding and the nails that held it on, were loaded on the lighters. The tugs with their load departed in the dark for unknown ports. During the next day, the sheriff from Sault Ste Marie, Michigan, located them, stuck in the ice in Canadian waters near St. Joseph Island. As they had crossed the International Boundary, he was powerless, particularly as one of the mill owners threatened him with a gun. That sheriff went home. When the ice broke up, the tugs and lighters moved down the North Channel, arriving at Moiles Harbour on John Island where the mill was hastily re-assembled and where it sawed logs for many years. Some remnants of this mill were still visible for the venturesome yachtsman to see in this pretty harbour in the 1970s, as I can attest.

By no means was all the timber hauled out onboard ship. Tremendous rafts were made up and pulled by tugs all the way to Buffalo where in 1890, there were 132 lumber firms sawing the logs into lumber, milling to shape and marketing. The loads hauled to Detroit, Buffalo, Chicago, Sandusky and Cleveland were apt to be square timber, rough planks, shingles, lathe, fence posts, barrel staves, telegraph poles and even tanbark. At first, the products of the forest

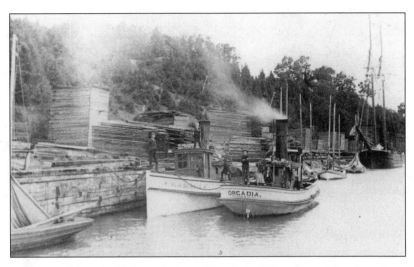

Two tugs, the Seibold *(1901), later named the* Theonli, *and the* Orcadia
*(1901) were typical of those built at the Marlton Shipyards in Goderich.
Frequently, they were used to tow log booms from the northern ports along
Georgian Bay and north of Manitoulin Island to the local sawmills, where
the logs were cut into lumber to meet local demands and for shipment by rail.
The schooner in the background is loading lumber. The other sailing vessels
are typical of those found along the shores of Lake Huron.* Courtesy of the
Huron County Museum.

would be carried in vessels with large timber-ports, built into the
stern, allowing the long squared timber to be loaded directly into the
hold. The hold would be filled solid, as close to the deck as possible.
Then huge wedges were driven between the timber and the deck
beams to help the deck support 12-foot high loads of additional
timber, gunwale to gunwale, from foremast to mizzen. The sails were
fitted with a "lumber reef," raising the boom to clear the timber piles,
rather than reefing the sails down as was the usual fashion. The hard-
working sailors who brought the ship into port and sailed her away
again were pressed into duty to load and unload, frequently helped by
other stevedores who took on the name of "lumber shovers."

Eventually it was not economical to ship timber in this manner.
The schooners were getting old. The pretty lines and ship-shape spars
and rigging could not be economically maintained when schedules
depended on wind and weather. Spars were cut down, bowsprits

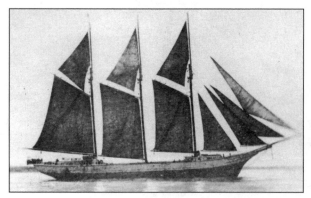

The J.T. Wing *was a regular visitor to Goderich Harbour and other ports along the lakes. She carried logs from the north in her holds and stacked high on her large open decks, taking them to mills in southern Ontario to meet the pressing needs of the lumber trade. As the age of sail came to an end, so too did the voyages of grand vessels like the* Wing. *Her last load was carried to the Goderich docks in the mid-1930s.* Courtesy of Bill Linfield.

removed, and steam tugs would tow four or five of these timber barges, at times assisted by the limited remaining sail area. Nor was this fate restricted to the timber droghers. It became the destiny of the majority of the old sail craft.

It is fascinating to examine art depicting some of the early craft and compare this with photos of ships taken during the last days of commercial sail on the lakes. The ships had become "scruffy" to say the least, with deep bruises and scrapes caused by battering of ice and working among the large and heavy log booms. They may have looked a sorry state, but they still represented the glory of a vanishing fleet.

It was customary for many of the timber droghers to carry a team of horses on deck. In port, the team was harnessed to tackle for lifting and shifting the loads of big timbers, both loading and unloading. Their care was entrusted to a youth, the lowest in the hierarchy on board, known as the horseboy. Rafts as huge as two million feet of oak, buoyed up by a million feet of pine as long as 1,000 feet and over a hundred feet wide, would be hauled by two or more tugs. They often took 16 days or more to get from Bay City to Buffalo or from Georgian Bay to a Lake Huron port. They were a menace to navigation, being rarely properly lit. In 1897, the steam passenger ship, *Cambria*, plowed into a raft of telephone poles and was wrecked.

An out of the ordinary delivery scheme was devised by the Wiarton firm of Seaman and Newman who contracted to deliver half a million feet of timber from the Bruce to Sault Ste. Marie in 1891, for use in the construction of the canal on the Canadian side. A "raft" was assembled, 175 feet long, 25 to 30 feet wide and some 12 feet thick, of solid hemlock, all fastened together at the ends with long steel rods. It was virtually a solid wooden barge in itself and was towed by a steam tug all the way to the Sault. Some six million feet of hemlock were hauled in this manner over a six-year period and only once did a violent storm cause any serious loss.

The Grand Haven rig evolved in the lumber trade. Tradition has it that a master of a three-masted schooner from that port was forced to have his mainmast taken out due to rot. He found the vessel sailed under the remaining mizzen and foresails quite as well as she had with the two additional sails on the foremast. She had the added advantage of more space for storing timber on deck, and the idea was copied by other ship owners.

In 1861, a large barque was built especially for the lumber trade by interests in Cleveland, and named the *City of Chicago*. She could carry half her load, a dead weight of almost 400 tons on deck. Having no foreboom, as a barque, there was more room to carry lumber on deck, forward of the mainmast. She proved to be highly profitable as the loading and unloading time was greatly reduced.

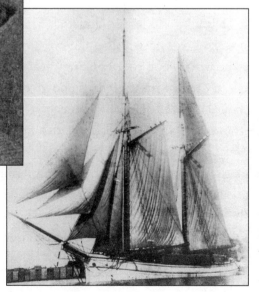

Captain John MacDonald of Goderich was skipper of the Azov *of Hamilton (108 x 23.7 feet, a 10-foot draught) a large schooner that hauled lumber. The Azov is shown under sail in 1902.* Photo of Captain MacDonald is courtesy of Donald Bert MacAdam, owner and former operator of MacDonald Marine. Photo of the *Azov of Hamilton* is courtesy of the Bruce County Museum & Cultural Centre: A968.022.001.

A three-masted barque, the *Sarah Ann March*, was built at Port Hope in 1854 and fitted with lumber ports in the stern. After extensive use she had been so strained by heavy deck loads that she had to be frapped or corsetted by passing heavy chains around the hull and tightening them with turnbuckles on deck. She carried on in this way for many years and doubtless was not alone in receiving such treatment.

John MacDonald was the patriarch of a long line of mariners who accomplished many nautical feats at Goderich and other Lake Huron ports. He was the skipper of the *Azov of Hamilton*, a large sailing schooner that hauled lumber between Lake Michigan and the Port of Goderich. The *Azov* was wrecked in a storm in late 1911 while on return to Goderich, on the American side of Lake Huron, east of Pointe aux Barques. Rather than land on a foreign shore, Captain John, his woman cook (his daughter Ettie Drennan) and crew of six men abandoned ship and rowed the ship's yawl back home to Goderich in a gruelling ordeal. They landed about six miles north of their intended destination.

The *Azov*, her deck awash, drifted across the lake and finally came to rest at McGregor's Point near Port Elgin. Her wreckage and anchor were discovered in 1956 by descendant Bruce MacDonald and a friend Allan MacDonald (not related), after a lengthy search for her remains. The anchor currently adorns one of the waterfront parkettes along the bluff overlooking Goderich Harbour. The MacDonalds – generations of them – are best known for their lifesaving efforts and rescue work along the shorelines near this port. In more modern times, *Captain John* was the name given to a small wooden work tug built by descendants of the same family in the last shipbuilding efforts to take place at Goderich Harbour in the 1940s.

The pine forests were stripped of their best trees, and the smaller trees and slash were fired to clear the land for farming, leaving the countryside a burned-out wasteland. The white pine forests of Michigan virtually disappeared in a few decades. The lumbering activity was accompanied by numerous tragic forest fires, some of which were caused by lumbermen burning slash, others by the settlers in their efforts to clear the land for agricultural purposes. Many hundreds of thousands of acres of fine timber were completely destroyed. On the same night that the great Chicago fire started, a fire swept across much of the state from the shores of Lake Michigan to the shores of Lake Huron. Holland and Manistee, in Michigan on the eastern shore of Lake Michigan, were virtually destroyed along with smaller communities and many farmsteads. Thousands of people were made homeless, some driven into the lake for refuge from the heat. One family and the children of another drifted for several days, finally arriving at Goderich on the Canadian shore.

And that was only one of many fires. In another, in September 1881, one hundred and twenty-five lives were lost, 3400 buildings destroyed and 1,800 square miles of Michigan burned over.

Novelists have frequently pictured the life of the woodsman with an aura of romance. From our point of view today, it certainly was a life of extreme hardships, wasteful not only of timber but of men. The woodsmen were as rough and wild a group of men as ever congregated anywhere, and their lives were apt to be hard and short. The shanties or "cambooses," as they were called, in which they lived all winter, were log buildings caulked with moss. They were built with the intention of lasting only a few years, and then the men would move on to greener fields. The walls were lined with two tiers of bunks with balsam boughs for mattresses. At eight or nine in the evening, the men all piled in, head first and feet towards the fire, gar-nering the heat from one or more pot-bellied stoves. Sometimes they were so crowded they had to roll over in unison at the call of "Spoons."

Breakfast was served before daybreak. The cook was the first to rise and would wake the men with the call, "Roll out!" or "Daylight in the swamp!" or even more picturesque language, at four or five in the morning.

Meals were hardy and filling – baked beans, bread, strong tea, for breakfast. The men who worked near the camp might come in for a noon meal and the cook would provide the others with a portable kitchen on a sleigh. Supper was the big meal. Salt pork, pea soup, bread and potatoes supplemented by game or fish, on occasion, would be followed by pie, cake or doughnuts and coffee. Meals were eaten in total silence for it was discovered quite early that discussion all too often started arguments. Arguments between men armed with a sharp knife and fork could be disastrous. For the same reason, liquor was not allowed in the camps, but that is not to suggest that it never got there.

Although life in the camp may have been hard and without much variety, the men made up for it when they got to town. Decked out in their best garments, multicoloured, plaid mackinaws in red, green or blue, tasselled caps, broad red sashes and heavy lumberjack boots, they were all set for carousing and brawling, vying with each other to spend their money as quickly as possible, to "blow their stakes."

Every saloon in town did a roaring business. Various writers have described the men as they hit town. Sir Richard Bonnycastle, in 1848, described their interests as "…the fiddle, the female, and the fire-water."[2] Holbrook listed their needs as "booze, bawds and battle."[3] Harlan Hatcher writes that the only thing they wanted came in bottles or corsets.[4] By any words, it remains the same. Each town had its street of saloons. In Bay City, the street was named "Hell's Half Mile." Saginaw had 32 saloons in the space of a few blocks. But statistics do not tell the whole story and it can never be relived. The immense forests are gone and along with them, the lumberjacks, the timber droghers and the seamen who were their crew.

As a personal note here, I still remember visiting one of these camps in Northern Ontario. I was a youngster of perhaps 13 years, travelling with my father as he made his "occasional" pastoral call to the woodsmen. He was a Protestant minister and we lived in a town some thirty miles away. The year would have been around 1935. I have forgotten most of the visit, but not the meal provided to my father and me. A healthy stew, lots of meat and vegetables, constituted the main course. On top was one or two thick slices of bread and on top of that, a large piece of apple pie. Even a healthy youngster who had no appetite problems could not manage more than a part of that fare.

CHAPTER 20

Other Commercial Sail,
Ore Carriers and Stone Hookers

THE EARLIEST MINING ON THE SHORES of the Great Lakes goes back long before the arrival of the white man and relates to the deposits an the south shore of Lake Superior where copper was found in the metallic state. This rare occurrence, one of very few in the world where copper naturally appears in this fashion, was used by the Natives centuries ago for making axe heads, spear points and arrow heads. In 1664, Pierre Boucher, an early French explorer, wrote of finding ingots of pure copper.[1] One natural ingot discovered in 1848 is reported to have weighed six tons. The first copper brought out was in 1687, but attempts to exploit the find at that time were stalled by the Iroquois Wars. In 1727, La Ronde made plans to mine the deposits and built a little vessel of 25 tons at Sault Ste Marie, the first sailing ship on Superior. He had great plans for the copper find including settlements and agriculture, but again the Indian wars disrupted the plans. In 1767, British explorers re-discovered the mineral and a company was formed in England to work it. In 1769, another vessel was built at the Sault, a 40-ton sloop, built by Alexander Baxter. High purity silver was also found by these explorers and mining started off with great expectations but fizzled out a few years later.

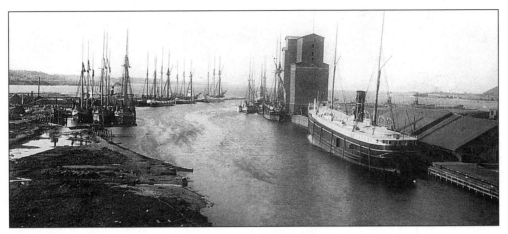

The steamer in the Owen Sound Harbour is a CPR freighter. The sailing schooners are grain carriers loading bulk cargo from the elevator. These vessels were from Great Lakes ports, especially Chicago. Courtesy of the Grey Bruce Image Archives.

The next explorer to report finding ore was Henry Schoolcraft,[2] in 1820, but the first practical copper mining on the shores of Lake Superior was not carried out until 1844. Mining continued until around 1875 when it had reached the point where the Michigan mines were turning out 80% of the nations' needs.

Iron mining started about the same time in the 1800s. The first small vessel to arrive at the Carp River had to anchor off and unload onto Ripley's Rock, at 1,000 feet from shore. From here the cargo was

The original is a 1900 coloured postcard of the Kingston (Ontario) waterfront, roughly from the end of Princess Street to Queen Street. The view is from the top of one of the grain elevators in the harbour. An unidentified two-masted schooner lies alongside a wharf and a pile of coal. The whiter stone building in the middle left of the picture is City Hall. Courtesy of Walter Lewis, Maritime History of the Great Lakes webmaster.

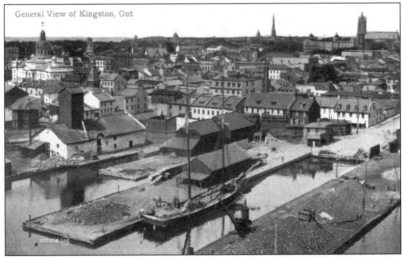

General View of Kingston, Ont

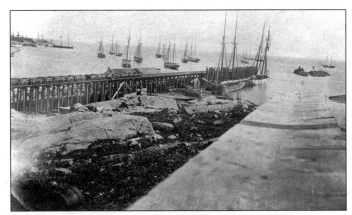

Loading ore at Marquette, Michigan, 1863. Courtesy of the Marquette Historical Society Inc.

transferred to the mainland in small boats or else floated in to the beach. Similarly, loading was accomplished by bringing barrels of ore out to the vessel in small boats or barges. At the Sault, all ore and supplies had to be off-loaded and transported by land over the mile-long portage, then loaded up again. This backbreaking job continued until the Sault Canal was opened in 1855.

At Marquette, Michigan (on the south shore of Lake Superior), docks were soon built out into the lake, some of which were short-lived due to severe Superior storms. Now the schooners could come along-side and the ore be conveyed on board by wheelbarrows and dumped on deck. It was rarely put down below at first, due to the difficulty of unloading from the hold. It would take a gang of 20 to 30 men from three to five days to load 100 to 300 tons of ore onto a ship. The men were reported to receive 25 cents a day for this back-breaking labour.

In 1857, trestlework and a pier were built there – the first iron ore "pocket" loading dock. The ore was brought out in little four-wheeled cars pulled by mules over a strap railway[3] and dumped into the pockets and then fed in through wooden chutes into the vessel. At first the captains objected as they feared that the ore, falling for such a distance (25 feet), would punch holes in the bottoms of their little wooden ships. Probably it would not punch actual holes, but there were several cases reported of sprung frames.

In 1855, the brig *Columbia* sailed from Marquette with a load of 132 tons of ore and was the first vessel to carry ore through the

Below: The St. Joseph Wharf, stretching out into Lake Huron about ten miles north of Grand Bend, was built by Narcisse Cantin to service his planned-for but never-achieved canal connecting Lakes Erie and Huron. Right: Shown here is the schooner, the Julia Larsen, *unloading freight, including barrels of petroleum, at the wharf. A number of the local folk are visiting the dockside.* Both images courtesy of the Huron County Museum.

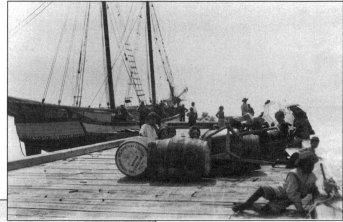

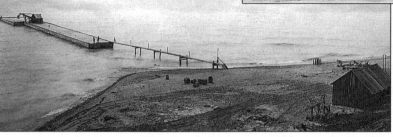

Sault Canal, all the way to Cleveland. Ninety-one feet long and of 177 tons burthen, she had been built at Sandusky in 1842.

As part of the grandiose plans of the Great Lakes and Atlantic Canal and Power Company Limited to establish a "Great Lakes to Ocean Route," a 43-nautical mile canal with one lock to lift vessels the nine-foot difference between Lake Erie and Lake Huron, was proposed in 1919. It was to be built from Port Stanley on Lake Erie and enter Lake Huron at St. Joseph, just north of Grand Bend. In preparation for this venture, Narcisse Cantin laid out plans for a new city at this location and constructed a dock along the shore. He actually built a grand hotel and some of the preliminary buildings and factories to demonstrate his commitment with real investment in its future potential. While the venture never did succeed, the dock was busy offloading freight and providing dockage for fishing boats for many years in the first quarter of the 20th century.

Hundreds of small sailing craft were used in the hauling of Lake Superior ores. They continued in use up to about the turn of the

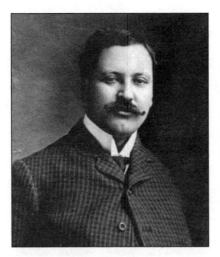

Narcisse M. Cantin (1870–1940), a visionary, raised millions for the building of a shipping canal to connect Lake Huron to Lake Erie. Despite his fundraising efforts, all came to an end when some potential investors lost interest in the project following the outbreak of the First World War. Courtesy of Paul Carroll, from the late Napoleon Cantin.

century, though by that time they were almost all used as "hookers," and were hauled five or six in a row behind steam tugs. The term applied to ore carriers and lumber carriers and would appear to have been used on Lake Superior only. At times small sails were used to help the train of hookers on its way. An example of a schooner being hauled is found in the story of the steam barge *Bruno* and the *Louisa*,

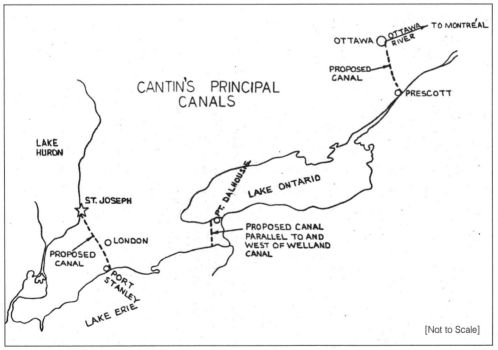

Narcisse Cantin envisioned other canals. When the St. Joseph project came to an end, he moved on to promote canals in Quebec along what would become the St. Lawrence Seaway. Courtesy of Paul Carroll.

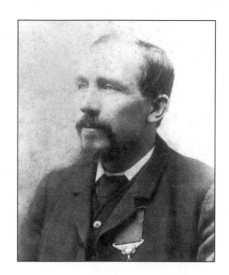

Captain William Babb of Goderich wearing his US Congress Silver medal for bravery, awarded for rescuing the crew of an American ship, 1885. The medal is on display at the Huron County Museum. Courtesy of the Huron County Museum.

a three-masted schooner, both owned by Captain George P. Magann of Toronto. Both vessels were loaded with coal from Cleveland and bound for Toronto. "We left Cleveland at 10 a.m. on November 1 [1890], coal-laden, and had a good trip until reaching Thunder Bay Tuesday morning when we encountered a terrific gale from the southeast, accompanied by a very heavy sea... ." The *Bruno* was towing the *Louisa*. On Wednesday, November 11, these vessels were wrecked on Magnetic Reef, between Cockburn and Manitoulin islands. Captain Alexander Peters of Toronto, captain of the *Bruno*, and the crews of both ships narrowly escaped drowning.[4]

Stories of shipwrecks on the Great Lakes are legion and have been captured in music, legend and countless tales. Along with these stories are ones extolling the bravery of men who rescue those caught in shipwrecks. One such person was William Babb of Goderich, the distinguished recipient of the US Congress Silver medal in "testimony of heroic deeds in saving lives from the perils of the sea" on the American schooner, the *A.C. Maxwell*, in a storm on Lake Huron on December 9, 1885, along with other members of the Goderich Life Saving Brigade. Babb was the commander for the Goderich Lifeboat Station at the time. Lifeboat stations were located at every significant harbour along the Great Lakes, positioned to perform search and rescue operations for ships wrecked near the shore that had tried and failed

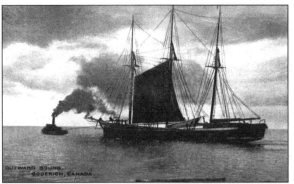

The Kahaden, a three-masted schooner, is being hauled out to meet the evening breezes as she sets out from Goderich on Lake Huron, under tow by small wooden tug. The undated postcard image was a colourized rendition to show the blazing colours of the setting sun. Courtesy of the Bayfield Archives.

to enter the safety of harbours of refuge during storms. In the days of sail, these lifesaving crews played an enormously important role in rescue work, and saved countless lives in their volunteer work. Captain Babb also operated the Ocean House Hotel during the mid-1880s in Lowertown at Goderich Harbour. It was located adjacent to the artesian mineral springs, then touted for their amazing healing qualities, and which attracted patrons from far afield to stay in his hotel and bathe in these restorative waters.

There was an entirely different type of boat on Lake Ontario, one that took the name "stone hooker." These were very common from the Credit River to as far east as Oshawa from the 1830s, until just after the First World War. The industry rose from the need for heavy stone for foundations of large homes and public buildings and were essential until quality Portland cement became available. Large blocks of shale were found along the shore in water shallow enough for harvesting. In use, the stone hooker would anchor as close to the shore as possible, usually in from six to twelve feet of water. Men, in small flat bottom scows, would gather the "stones" from the bottom by hooking with a two-pronged fork with the tines made at right angles to the handle. The stones would be loaded into the barge, then transferred to the "hooker" and carried to Toronto, or wherever they were needed. At the height of the industry, as many as 5,000 tons of stone would be harvested from the bottom of Lake Ontario in a year. A ton totalled 216 cubic feet and would bring from $3.00 to $5.00.

They were not pretty vessels, some not much more than a box, slab-sided, almost flat-bottomed, square-ended, but fitted with two or more centreboards. Nearly all were schooner-rigged. They ranged from 20 to 100 tons and carried crib stone, gravel, building stone, pavers and sand and occasionally grain or cordwood, and always under sail. One could never rate them as fast or seaworthy boats, but they ranged all of Lake Ontario and sailed to windward after a fashion though they were at their best downwind. Each year, in the Toronto area, a race was held and from the stories told, even racing in an ugly stone hooker scow could be exciting.

Epilogue

I can't help feeling lonesome for the ships that have gone,
For the sight of Huron sunsets and the hours before the dawn,
And the white sails pullin' stoutly to a warm and steady draft,
And the smell o' roastin' coffee, and the watches run aft.
I'd like to ship offshore again upon some tidy barque,
And sing a sailor shanty in the windy starry dark,
Or first a clewed-up tops'l in a black south-easter roar,
But what's the use of wishing; for them days will come no more.[1]

I STARTED RESEARCHING FOR THIS BOOK in 1972 when I was navigating a desk in an office tower in downtown Chicago. It was a spare-time project and conducted while running a bureaucratic type of job, sailing Lake Michigan and keeping the family content and the children in university. By the time of my retirement in 1984, the research was essentially finished and a draft manuscript prepared, but no publisher in sight.

With no immediate prospects at the time, I decided to sail for a few years. The Great Lakes were too small for me so I headed for the Atlantic and Europe and wherever my wife Jean and I fancied, for as long as it brought us both happiness.

My sailing career ended in 2000, after sailing some 25,000 miles, visiting and exploring every European country that had a salt-water coastline and crossing wherever canals and rivers could take us in Europe. Health problems brought this adventure to an end when I reached my early eighties, but it was wonderful while it lasted.

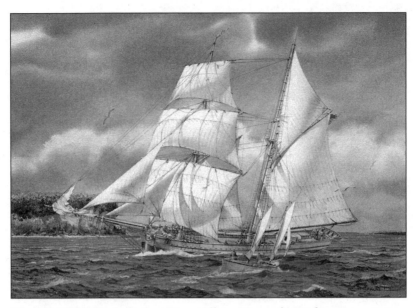

The Alvin Clark *was built at Truago (later Trenton), Michigan, in 1846. A "packet schooner" of 218 tons, 106' x 25' x 9', she sank during a storm just off Chambers Island in Green Bay, Wisconsin, in 1864. In 1967, a fisherman snagged his nets on her mast – the* Alvin Clark *standing upright in 110 feet of water. Two men, Frank Hofman and a Mr. Derusha, raised her in 1969. A remarkable treasure trove of artefacts, she was towed into Marinette, Michigan, where she was opened for tourist visits. In spite of very serious efforts to have her restored, they were unsuccessful and the vessel soon rotted away. I had the privilege of being one of those tourists and of standing on her deck and imagining the spray flying. A sad finish for a proud ship! Charles L. Peterson, artist.*

But getting back to the manuscript, I found that my word processor/computer of the 1970s and 80s was not compatible with systems of the year 2000. To start with, the manuscript had to be scanned, page by page, and converted into a new word processing program by a friend, then brought up to date. And then there have been the inimitable corrections and amendments.

So, the book is a longstanding effort covering 32 years, but it never was allowed to get in the way of my sailing. If it brings you a fraction of the pleasure that the researching and writing have brought me, then it has been worthwhile. I hope it will inspire you

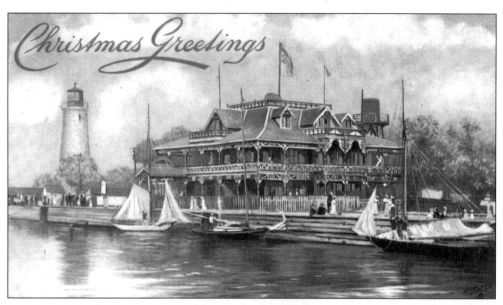

Even as the heyday of commercial sail had started to decline, the era of pleasure sailboats began its ascension. Small vessels, previously designed for commercial use, had been redesigned to accommodate the desires of wealthier citizens who found great pleasure, along with new social status, as members of distinguished yacht clubs found along the lakes. While most of these associations were found in large urban areas, many smaller clubs were formed around the lakes. Today, yachts persist everywhere for persons of a range of economic levels, albeit not as formal as the "Royal Yacht Clubs" of yesteryear. This photograph of the Royal Hamilton Yacht Club and its buildings in Hamilton, Ontario, is a treasured relic from those earlier days. The original is a hand-coloured oilette, printed in England around 1900. The RHYC buildings burned on September 18, 1915. Postcard photograph courtesy of Janet Forjan-Freedman.

to borrow or perhaps even to buy some of the books in my bibliography and to pursue the subject much further.

By 1890 the peak of commercial sail had passed. A few continued to operate, primarily in the lumber trade, but by 1920 sight of any commercial schooner was a rarity indeed. There is no doubt we have lost "something" with the passing into history of commercial sail. To those who love the Great Lakes and sailing on them (or just watching), it is a bit "something" and precious. The skills of the shipwrights and artificers who designed and built the big vessels, and the skill, bravery and even masochism of those who worked the boards, for long hours and at times in great danger, is too important to our history to be lost.

I've sailed a 128-foot schooner in the Caribbean and been both a tourist/guest and a "pully-hauley" crew. It was only a holiday, 60 years ago, but I'll never forget it. The experience of youth on Toronto's Brigantines and other sail-training vessels around the world is invaluable in building character and a respect for our naval history. All such experiences should be encouraged.

The Great Lakes are both an historical and a natural treasure. We need to care for them.

Appendix A:
Brief Biographies of Featured Artists

Duncan Macpherson (1924-1993)

DUNCAN IAN MACPHERSON was born to Scottish parents in Toronto in 1924. He attended North Toronto Collegiate Institute and, briefly, Central Technical School. In 1942, he enlisted in the Canadian Air Force, serving until 1945 in England where his cartoons and sketches soon appeared in the Canadian Armed Services' Second World War newspaper, *The Maple Leaf*.

He studied at the London Polytechnic (Holborn) at the Boston Museum School of Fine Art, and at the Ontario College of Art. He began his career as a freelance illustrator with the *Montreal Standard*, *Maclean's* and other publications. In 1958, he joined the *Toronto Star* as editorial cartoonist. He drew his last cartoon only two months before his untimely death in 1993.

His combination of humour and artistic ability created brilliant cartoons. He has been recognized by the public and his peers as Canada's best cartoonist. He received the Order of Canada, The Queen Elizabeth Jubilee Medal, the Canada Council Molson Award, the Canadian Royal Academy Medal, was made a fellow of the Ontario College of Art, won the National Newspaper Award for Cartooning six times and was named to the News Hall of Fame. Collections of his cartoons are at the National Archives of Canada, the Boston Public Library, the Art Gallery of Ontario and the Toronto Daily Star.

In his travels for the *Star*, he drew on-the-spot news items of world events that sent him to Cuba, the Clayton Ruby trial in Texas,

US political conventions, France, China and Russia. During four summers he crossed Canada, producing in watercolour, drawings and pastels, his portrait of Canada entitled "Macpherson's Canada." On holiday, he would paint watercolours on the spot or bring sketches home to complete in his studio. He had been a long-time summer resident of Beaverton on Lake Simcoe and a reduced cartoon schedule in 1980 allowed him to reside there permanently.

He painted a masterful series of six early Scottish historical figures he called the "Celtic Hexagon," which were purchased by James C. Baillie and donated to the Beaverton Public Library.

Alexander McNeilledge

Born to a Greenock, Scotland, seafaring family on November 8, 1791, Alexander McNeilledge had become a cabin boy aboard his father's ship, the *Pandora*, by the age of nine. He worked his way up the chain of command, and, by the age of 31, had become the captain of the brig, the *Saunders*. McNeilledge sailed mainly in the East India and China trades, taking him to ports all around the world where he was involved in many daring adventures, including blockade running, smuggling gold and outwitting pirates.

His first trip to Norfolk County came in 1829 when he landed at the mouth of the Lynn River to visit his brother at Dover Mills (Port Dover). Captain McNeilledge quit the seafaring life in June of 1830 and decided to stay in Dover with his wife, Mary Ann Thum, as a bookkeeper for his brother's endeavours. By 1936 he had changed his avocation again and bought land to the north of Port Dover. However, having no interest in farming, he left that to his wife and son while he made daily trips to the harbour and became involved in many operations around the port. His most famous contribution to the lake came during the 1840s when he produced charts and maps for navigating Lake Erie. Many were the first ever done for the area and were considered an invaluable resource for the vessels travelling the unforgiving lake.

Captain McNeilledge recorded many historical important events in his diary, which he kept for over 40 years. His entries dealt with countless topics, including the coming of steamers to the harbour and the building and launching of numerous from the shipyards. He died on August 20, 1874.

Charles L. Peterson

After service in World War II, Charles Peterson studied at Chicago's Art Institute and graduated from the American Academy of Art. He earned a BA at Marietta College, an MFA at Ohio University and pursued study at the University of Wisconsin. Thereafter, he enjoyed a distinguished twenty-year career as Professor of Art, including fifteen years as head of the Art Department at Marietta College. In 1973, Professor Peterson moved with his family to Ephraim, Wisconsin, and took up a new career as full-time painter, a vocation in which he soon established a national reputation.

Initially, Peterson became widely known through his illustrations for *Wooden Boat*, *Sail*, *Cruising World* and other boating magazines. In 1987, he was invited to show his work at the prestigious Mystic Maritime Museum Gallery's International Competitions where, in 1991 and again in 1992, he won the coveted Thomas Hoyne Award.

In 1998, The White Door Publishing Company began national distribution of Peterson's "Memories Collection" and his "Maritime Collection" of signed, limited edition prints, widening the circle of enthusiastic collectors of his work. This popularity grew so quickly that as early as 1992, *US Art* magazine began listing him among the nation's top ten most popular artists in the print industry. White Door published his first book, *Of Time and Place* in 1994 and his second book, *Reflections* in 2001.

In 2006, Peterson won the prestigious Museum Purchase Award at the 27th Annual International Mystic Seaport Gallery Exhibition in New London, Connecticut. The painting is titled *The Grace Deering Arrives in Boston.*

O.K. "Ozzie" Schenk (1914-2002)

Born and educated in Nova Scotia, Ozzie Schenk graduated from the Nova Scotia College of Art and Design in 1933, did post-graduate studies at the Central School of Art and Design in London, England, in 1936 and started his career there.

In 1939, he was commissioned in the RNVR and served at sea in the Second World War in the Royal Navy. In 1946, he returned to Canada and was employed as Art Director by several of Toronto's best known advertising agencies. He retired in 1980 from Rous, Mann and Brigdens Ltd. where he had been serving as Senior Design Consultant.

He served in many positions in the art professional societies yet still found time and energy for altruistic service. He was President of the Canadian Save the Children Fund for a time. He served on the Board and was Past Vice-President and Honorary Life Member of Toronto Brigantine, a sail-training program for youth on the Great Lakes, whose objectives are summarized in their slogan "Bringing character through adventure."

Of course he was an enthusiastic sailor all his life, sailing from the Royal Canadian Yacht Club. He was an active member of the "Provincial Marine of 1812," a group of enthusiastic model builders and amateur historians.

Ozzie was elected to the Ontario Society of Artists in 1982, the Canadian Society of Painters in Water Colour in 1989, the Canadian Society of Marine Artists in 1990 and the Royal Canadian Academy of Arts in 1994 and was a member of the Arts and Letters Club of Toronto. He has received many awards and citations. Over four hundred of his watercolours hang in corporate and private collections in Canada and the United States.

Ozzie Schenk is best known for his marine watercolours and acrylics, which he rendered with an understanding and authority based on long familiarity with the sea and coastal environment.

Appendix B: Chronology

1615-1760	Period of exploration and control by the French
1678	La Salle builds four small ships at Fort Frontenac (Kingston)
1679	La Salle builds the *Griffon* and makes the first voyage in the Upper Lakes.
1726	The French build two schooners at Fort Frontenac
1743-1756	The French build more ships at Fort Frontenac and start building at Niagara.
1754	The British start building a fleet at Oswego
1756	The French attack Oswego and capture the British vessels.
1758	The British capture Fort Frontenac.
1760	The British defeat French in the St. Lawrence River. The Canadas become British.
1763	The Peace of Paris ends the Seven Years War (Feb. 10).
1762	The British build their first ships on the Upper Lakes at Navy Island
1764	The first ships were built at Detroit.
1777	The Provincial Marine is established. Immigration, fur trading, shipbuilding and other commerce grow rapidly.
1789	The schooner, *Nancy*, is built at Detroit.
1783	The Treaty of Paris ends the American Revolution.
1796	The first United States armed vessel, the *Detroit*, is built at Detroit.
1804	The first lighthouse on the Great Lakes begins operation at York.
1808	The first United States Navy vessel, the *Oneida*, is built at Oswego.

1812	June 18: United States declares war against Britain and Canada.
1812	July 12: American forces, led by General William Hull, invade Canada at Sandwich. After ravaging and looting farms and homes for sixty miles around, he withdraws the American army on August 7 under cover of darkness.
1812	July 17: British capture Michilimackinac.
1812	August 16: the British, under Sir Isaac Brock, capture Detroit.
1812	October 13: the American forces are defeated at Queenston Heights. Sir Isaac Brock is killed.
1813	April 27: the Americans capture York, burning and looting buildings. Stores and cannon intended for Robert Barclay at Fort Malden are captured. The *Sir Isaac Brock* is burned in the stocks.
1813	May 16: Sir James Lucas Yeo arrives at Kingston as Commodore of the Fleets on the Great Lakes.
1813	May 27: American forces capture Fort Erie.
1813	May 29: The British under Sir James Yeo, attack Sacket's Harbor and withdraw without accomplishment.
1813	June 24: the Provincial Marine is taken over by the Royal Navy.
1813	August 8: the *Hamilton* (USN) and the *Scourge* (USN) are hit by a severe squall and sink off the mouth of the Niagara River.
1813	September 10: the Battle of Lake Erie gives victory over the Upper Lakes to the American navy.
1813	September 25: Sir James Yeo and Commodore Isaac Chauncey fight a brief but vicious battle off Burlington (sometimes referred to as "the Burlington Races."
1813	September 26: the British forces withdraw from Detroit.
1813	September 27: Americans invade across the Detroit River and General Proctor retreats from Fort Malden.

1813	October 5: American army advances up the Thames River to Moravian Town where they defeat the British. Tecumseh is killed.
1813	December 10: American army retreats from the Niagara Peninsula, burning Newark as they go.
1813	December 19: British capture Fort Niagara and burn Lewiston and Buffalo in retaliation.
1814	April 11: the Treaty of Fontainebleau settles the Napoleonic War.
1814	May 6: the British under Sir James Yeo attack Oswego and carry off some stores but leave much more behind.
1814	July 3: the British are defeated and lose Fort Erie again.
1814	July 20: the Americans destroy the remains of Fort St. Joseph.
1814	August 4: the American fleet under Captain Sinclair attack Michilimackinac but are repelled.
1814	August 12: the British capture the *Ohio* (USN) and the *Somers* (USN) while they are anchored at the entrance to the Niagara River.
1814	August 14: the *Nancy* is destroyed by the Americans at Wasaga.
1814	September 3&6: British forces capture the *Tigress* (USN) and the *Scorpion* (USN) near Drummond Island.
1814	In September, the *HMS St. Lawrence* is launched at Kingston
1814	December 24: the Treaty of Ghent is signed, ending the War of 1812.
1815	Commerce starts again and grows rapidly.
1816	The first steamship on the Great Lakes, the *SS Frontenac*, is launched at Bath, Ontario.
1818	The first lighthouses on the Upper Lakes at Buffalo and Erie commence operation.
1825	The Erie Canal is opened.
1825	First charts of Canadian waters are published.

1829	The first Welland Canal opens for traffic.
1855	The canal at Sault Ste. Marie links Lake Superior to the rest of the Great Lakes.
1870	The peak of commercial sailing, when over 2,000 ships are on the lists.
1889	Charting the American waters of the Great Lakes is completed and published.

Appendix C: Place Names

THE NAMES OF MANY HARBOURS and places have changed since the events recounted herein. In order to make it easier for the reader, the earlier names are given below along with the names by which they are known today.

L'Anse a la Construction: Maitland, Ontario

Black Rock: In the Niagara River at Buffalo, New York

Choueguen: Oswego, New York

Fort Malden: Amherstburg, Ontario

Matchedash: A bay at present-day Waubaushene, Ontario

Missilimackinac, Michilimackinac, Mackinac, Mich, (also pronounced Mackinaw): This applies to the fort, the straits, the island. (The first fort was at present day Mackinaw City and was built by the French in 1712. The British built a new one on Mackinac Island in 1781.)

Moy: Base for the North West Company, at Sandwich, Ontario (now Windsor)

Navy Island: A Canadian island in the Niagara River, above the Falls

Newark: Niagara-on-the-Lake, Ontario

Oswegatchie: Ogdensburg, New York

Presque Isle: Harbor at Erie, Pennsylvania

Presqu'île: Near Brighton, Ontario

Sandwich: Windsor, Ontario

Sacket's: in early writing, spelled Sackett's, Sacket's for the village as well as the harbor. Today is Sackets.

St. Mary's: Sault Ste. Marie, Ontario

York: Toronto, Ontario

Appendix D: Selected Glossary

Artificer: A craftsman, skilled workman, especially in the military.

Bateau: A small flat-bottomed boat rowboat used for transporting merchandise, e.g. furs, provisions or personnel.

Batten: A light piece of timber used to hold components together during assembly.

Block: A pulley of one or more sheaves (a grooved wheel commonly called a "shiv") through which lines are run.

Block and tackle: A combination of blocks and lines used for lifting heavy weights or exerting great force, e.g. to handle a large sail.

Brail: To furl up the sails to the mast or yards.

Brig: A vessel with two masts and square sails on both.

Brigantine: A vessel with two masts, square sails on the foremast and fore-and-aft sail on the mainmast.

Burthen or burden: The carrying capacity of a vessel or the weight of its cargo.

Capstan: An upright, spool shaped cylinder around which ropes or cables are wound and which is turned by removable wooden handles. Used for raising heavy weights such as timber frames, anchors, etc.

Caulk: The process of filling the joint between planks with oakum and pitch.

Ceiling: The planks which line and strengthen the hull; the inner walls and the "floor."

Chock: A triangular piece of timber used to join two futtocks together in making a frame.

Clamp: (i) A large beam attached to the inside of the ribs and supporting the deck beams; (ii) a tool somewhat like a large letter "G" with a screw to open or close it, used to hold timbers such as planks and ribs while they are being fitted and fastened.

Coak: A rectangular piece of oak about 2-4" thick, used in joining two components when using a scarf.

Compass timber: Piece of timber which had grown containing a curve, and used in shipbuilding for floors, ribs, knees, etc.

Corvette: A word with indefinite meaning over the years. A vessel smaller than a frigate. The word describes the purpose rather than a particular sail plan.

Deadwood: Timbers fitted between keel and stern post, or keel and stem, in order to fill and strengthen the area.

Draught: Plans for constructing a vessel. The depth of water a vessel requires.

Figurehead: A carved wooden figure attached at the head of the vessel and associated with the vessel's name.

Floor: A timber that crosses the keel and forms part of the frame.

Flotilla: A fleet of vessels, small or large, especially military vessels.

Fore-and-aft rig: A sail arrangement that uses sails set along the centreline rather than as square sails.

Forefoot: Essentially the same as the stem. See stem.

Frames: Any of the transverse structures that form the ribs of the ship's hull, also called ribs.

Frigate: Not a style of vessel, but rather denotes the size and armament, a medium-sized, fast and manoeuvrable warship

Futtock: Any of the upright curved timbers forming the ribs of a wooden vessel.

Gaff: A pole extending from the mast and supporting a sail.

Gin pole: A long pole fitted with a steel point at one end; usually used for propping up timbers.

Grapeshot. A cluster of small iron balls fired from a swivel mounted gun or cannon, usually directed against personnel.

Gunboat: A small vessel, rowing or sail, armed for close-in fight frequently with bow guns and swivels. Sometimes merchantmen were converted and armed for this use.

Gunwale: In the days of wooden ships, there was a row of heavy planks at the widest point in the hull, called the wales. They added strength to the gun deck. The heaviest was called the gunwale, or the main wale. In recent years it has come to mean the joint where the side of the hull meets the deck, usually reinforced by wood or metal.

Hanging knee: A piece of compass timber mounted vertically to the inside wall of the vessel, and used to support a deck beam.

Hulk: The hull of a vessel that has been taken out of service and is being used as a dormitory, a prison or a hospital ship.

Impressment: The practice of taking by force, landsmen and other sailors ashore, or even sailors from other ships, and forcing them to serve against their will.

Keel: The large timber extending along the entire length of the bottom of the vessel. The floors are positioned on this and they in turn form part of the frames.

Keelson: A large timber added over the floors, which with the keel makes up the backbone of the vessel, and gives it added strength.

Knee: A angled brace, in early shipbuilding, a piece of compass timber. Later steel knees became common. Knees were used to support and hold the deck beams to the bulwarks, the sides of the vessel.

Lateen: A triangular sail attached to a long pole (yard) hung at an angle from a short mast.

Lodging knee: A knee fitted horizontally to hold a deck beam in place.

Lofting: The practice of making "moulds" or thin wooden patterns for knees, futtocks, etc. taking information from the draughts.

Lugsail: A four-sided sail without a boom, attached to an upper yard hanging obliquely on the mast.

Mizzen: A fore-and-aft sail set on the aftmost mast, the mizzenmast.

Moccock: A birchbark container, shaped somewhat like a small canoe, used by the Natives to hold sugar for trade.

Moulds: Thin wooden patterns used to mark and shape the knees, futtocks, etc.

Oakum: A fibrous material made by unravelling old ropes. Used for caulking planks.

Rabbet: A groove cut in the edge of a timber so that the planks may be fitted into it to make a watertight joint.

Ribs: See frames.

Riband: A light piece of wood used as a temporary fastening, or used to "fair" a line of timbers.

Rider: Similar to a frame, mounted inside the vessel, across the keelson and to the walls to add extra strength to the hull.

Rigging: The lines that support the masts are standing rigging. The lines for handling the sails are running rigging.

Scarph or scarf: A method of joining timbers by bevelling each, overlapping, and fastening with treenails or steel bolts.

Schooner: A vessel of two or more masts, fitted with fore and aft sails.

Ship-rigged: A vessel with three or more masts and rigged with square sails.

Shipwright: A skilled woodworker, experienced in shipbuilding.

Shores: A pole or beam used to support a heavy component of a vessel under construction. Also used to support a vessel out of the water.

Slipway: A heavily built wooden structure. In building a vessel, the keel is laid on this.

Sloop: A fore-and-aft rigged vessel with one mast and one or more foresails.

Snow: A three-masted vessel, square-rigged on the fore and main masts and lateen-rigged on the mizzen. The mizzen is usually short and mounted very close to the mainmast.

Spalls: Temporary pieces of timber to hold components in place while being fastened.

Spanish windlass: A made-on-the-spot device for tightening a rope (for pulling or bending) by twisting it using a spindle and a lever.

Spar: A stout pole, used for the mast, yard etc, of a ship.

Spritsail: A four-sided sail with the upper, outer corner held out with a pole or sprit.

Square sail: A four-sided sail rigged to a yard suspended horizontally across the mast.

Square rigger: A three-masted ship with square sails on all masts.

Stem: An assembly of curved timbers that form the front of the hull. There are frequently other pieces forward of this, for strengthening and as "fashion pieces."

Sternpost: A heavy timber, nearly vertical at the very back end of the vessel. The rudder is attached to this.

Strake: A single row of outer planks, the length of the vessel.

Topsail schooner: A schooner with a square sail at the top of the foremast.

Treenail: A wooden peg, round or sixteen-sided, up to 1-3/4'' diameter, which is driven into a hole in the timbers in order to hold them together.

Tun: An archaic word meaning a cask, as used for wine, salted meat or flour etc. It held 252 wine gallons. The word defined the carrying capacity of the vessel by volume rather than by weight.

Wales: Several rows of heavy outer planks at the point of maximum beam of the vessel.

Notes

PART ONE: THE ERA OF FRENCH CONTROL ON
THE GREAT LAKES, 1678–1760

Chapter 1: The Beginning of Sail on Lake Ontario, 1678

1.   Louis Hennepin's memoirs were published in Paris on January 5, 1683, under the title *Description de la Louisiane, nouvellement découverte au sud-ouest de la Nouvelle-France par ordre du Roy*. The work had the most unqualified success and went through several editions and translations. Hennepin became a celebrity overnight and for a time his name was honoured until somewhere around 1687, for reasons that are not yet known, he suddenly fell into disgrace. Taken from the Dictionary of Canadian Biography Online (Jean-Roch Rioux) at http://www.biographi.ca/EN/ShowBio.asp?BioId=34963&query, accessed on Nov. 9, 2006.

2.   Pierre Pouchot, *Mémoires sur la Dernière Guerre de l'Amerique Septentrionale. entre la France et L'Angleterre: suivis d'observations dont plusiers sont relatives au théâtre actuel de la guerre, & de nouveau détails sur les moeurs & les usages des sauvages, avec des cartes topographiques*. Yvernon, France: 1781. Translated to English and edited by Hranklin B. Hough; printed for W.E. Woodward, 1866.

3.   New Amsterdam was the name given to the 17th century town that sprang up outside of Fort Amsterdam (1625) on Manhattan Island in the New Netherlands territory. The river (today's Hudson River) had been discovered, explored and charted by an expedition of the Dutch East India Company, captained by Henry Hudson, in 1609. The town acquired city status in 1653, but was unilaterally reincorporated as New York City by the British in 1665 (named after the Duke of York, later James II). Adapted from http://en.wikipedia.org/wiki/New°Amsterdam, accessed on Nov. 9, 2006.

4.   Louis de Buade de Frontenac et de Palluau is chiefly noted as the architect of French expansion in North America and the defender of New France against attacks by the Iroquois Confederacy and the English. He was born in May 1622. Louis XIII was his godfather. In the spring of 1672, Frontenac was appointed governor general of New France. Shortly after his arrival, Jean Talon, the Intendant, returned to France and Frontenac assumed the powers of the role of Intendant, an act that brought him into conflict with other officials and several leading families in the colony. Much to the annoyance of the merchant fur traders and the habitants of Montreal, Frontenac established a fur-trading post on Lake Ontario, at the mouth of the Cataraqui River where Kingston is today. The post became known as Fort Frontenac. Ultimately Frontenac's powers were curbed, a new Intendant was appointed and Frontenac's authority was restricted to military matters and supervision.

Frontenac became closely associated with Cavelier de la Salle to whom he gave assistance in establishing a monopoly of fur trade south of the Great Lakes. This brought Frontenac's associates into conflict with the Iroquois who were determined to seize the Ohio Valley for themselves. At the same time another threat to New France was developing in the north. In 1682, Frontenac was recalled to France, largely because of his continued wrangling with other officials. However, after France and England were once again at war, Frontenac was reappointed governor of New France in 1689 to replace the ailing incumbent. In January 1690 he mustered three war parties to ravage English border settlements, and succeeded in raising morale in New France. During the war years Frontenac greatly expanded the fur trade. New fur-trading posts were established in the west. Ultimately such activities led to ongoing conflict with the Iroquois, that were not resolved until the late 1690s. Frontenac died in 1707 and is buried at Quebec. Adapted from the Dictionary of Canadian Biography Online (W.J. Eccles) at http://www.biographi.ca/EN/ShowBio.asp?BioId=34218&query, accessed on Nov. 14, 2006.

5.   This translated and edited excerpt of a copy of the letter of authority from the King of France to La Salle, dated 1678, is taken from Frank H. Severance, *An Old Frontier of France: the Niagara Region and Adjacent Lakes under French Control*. Vol. II. New York: Dodd, Mead, 1917. It purports to be from French documents:

At St. Germain, May 12, 1678, the King and Councilor Colbert signed the license giving La Salle permission to pursue his explorations, or, in the words of the precious document, "to discover the western part of New France." "There is nothing," said Louis, "We have more at heart than the discover of that country, where there is a prospect of finding a way to penetrate as far as Mexico…These and other causes Us moving hereunto, We have permitted, and by these presents, signed by Our hand, do permit you to labor in the Discovery of the Western part of New France, and for the execution of this undertaking, to construct forts in the places you may think necessary, where of We will that you enjoy the same clauses and conditions as at Fort Frontenac…on condition, nevertheless, that you complete this enterprise within five years in default whereof, these presents shall be null and void; and that you do not carry on any trade with the Savages called Outaouacs and others who carry their beavers and peltries to Montreal; that you perform the whole at your expense and that of your associates, to whom we have granted, as a privilege, the trade in Cibola skins."

6.   La Motte de Lussiere seems to have joined with La Salle for the great adventure. It is likely he was a nobleman as La Salle trusted him enough to put him in charge of others. However, he only lasted a few months, returned to Montreal with eye trouble, then went back to France. La Motte seems to have been a sort of "partner" to share in proceeds of their venture. He and La Salle had a falling out, which may have been the cause of his leaving the expedition rather than the reported eye trouble.

7.   C.H.J. Snider, *Tarry Breeks and Velvet Garters: Sail on the Great Lakes Of America in War, Discovery and the Fur Trade Under the Fleur-de-Lys.* Toronto: Ryerson Press, 1958.

Chapter 2: The Building of the Griffon, 1679

1.   For more detailed information, see George Irving Quimby, *Indian Culture and European Trade Goods: the Archaeology of the Historic Period in the Western Great Lakes Region.* Madison, WI: University of Wisconsin Press, 1966; reprinted Westport, CT: Greenwood Press, 1978.

Chapter 3: The Voyage of the Griffon and the Loss: Where Is She Now?

1.   Pierre François-Xavier de Charlevoix (1682-1761) was born in France. A Jesuit priest and an explorer, he is most remembered for his explorations and his reports.

2.   Orie Vail, a local fisherman of Tobermory, Ontario, accidentally found remains of a wreck on Russell Island while fishing. He later became a

reporter/photographer for the *Toronto Telegram*, where he met C.H.J. Snider in the 1950s. They exchanged stories.

3. Rowley Murphy was an artist and an art instructor for the then Ontario Department of Education.

4. See Harrison John MacLean, *The Fate of the Griffon*. Toronto: Griffin House, 1974. McLean's work is not recommended as an authoritative text. He wrote about the Orie Vail find, which was later proven not to be the *Griffon*. To my mind there is no authoritative writing, nor any book which compares the various "finds", until this present book. The location of the *Griffon* is still, and may ever remain, a mystery.

5. For updated information, see www.lasalle-griffon.org, accessed on Nov. 22, 2006.

Chapter 4: The French Era Ends

1. Louis-Joseph de Montcalm, Marquis de Montcalm was born in France in 1712 and died in Quebec in 1759. At the age of nine, he began his military service as an ensign, but it would be 1732 before he began his active military career. After a short period of "peace-time" soldiering, Montcalm was appointed major-general to New France in 1756 where he was to be subordinate to the governor general of New France, Pierre de Rigaud Vaudreuil. Montcalm was to be responsible only for the discipline, administration and internal ordering of the army battalions. Inevitably, Montcalm and Vaudreuil would be at odds with one another. Dispatches of complaints were sent back to France.

In 1758, Montcalm was promoted to lieutenant-general, the second highest rank in the French army, much higher than a colonial governor general. This meant that Montcalm was given command of all the military forces in Canada and Vaudreuil was instructed to defer to him. In 1759, a series of errors on the part of the French and incredible luck for the British allowed the British forces under the command of General James Wolfe to have some 4,500 men on the Plains of Abraham, less than a mile from Quebec City. Montcalm chose to attack at once with the troops he had at hand, rather than wait for reinforcements. Both Montcalm and Wolfe were mortally wounded. Vaudreuil was obliged to capitulate to General Jeffery Amherst at Montreal the following September.

Historians have long been at odds in their assessment of Montcalm. Some have depicted him as the "gallant good and great Montcalm." Others find little good to say of him and hold him mainly responsible for the conquest of Canada. Adapted from http://www.biographi.ca/EN/ShowBio.asp?BioId=35664&query=, accessed on Nov. 29, 2006.

2.   Author's Note: The records are very incomplete. I was unable to find any mention of the *Halifax* after the French captured it and renamed it. One writer says that the French built a vessel at Cataraqui and named it the *Montcalm* in 1756. I suspect he is referring to the vessel captured at Oswego in 1756, but cannot confirm this.

3.   Pontiac, born sometime between 1712 and 1725, was war chief of the Ottawa from the Detroit area. Pontiac was described by those who saw him as a commanding, respected and highly intelligent leader. During the Seven Years War (the French and Indian War), Pontiac was loyal to the French. Following the surrender of Montreal in 1760, Native loyalties were divided. The British General Jeffrey Amherst (the commander-in-chief) forbade the customs of buying the Indians' good conduct with presents, and by 1762 the Natives had a scarcity of powder, lead and other commodities. Rumour of an Indian revolt became a full insurrection west of Lake Erie from 1763-64, with Pontiac a key leader. Ultimately, a peace mission sent by the English met with Pontiac in April 1765, bringing an end to the hostilities. Pontiac was murdered in 1769. From the Dictionary of Canadian Biography Online (Louis Chevrette) at http://www.biographi.ca/EN/ShowBio.asp?BioId=35719&query, accessed on Nov. 9, 2006.

4.   The American War of Independence (1775-1777) was essentially a colonial struggle against the political and economic policies of Great Britain. General George Washington built a new American army from scratch and generally controlled the countryside, while the British, with their naval superiority, were able to capture some coastal cities. The tide turned in 1777 when the war became more of a global conflict and France, with Spain and the Netherlands as allies, entered the war against Great Britain. The surrender of the main British army at Yorktown in 1781 effectively ended the land war, and the Treaty of Paris in 1783 recognized the independence of the United States.

As part of the conflict, Brigadier General Richard Montgomery marched north from Fort Ticonderoga and captured Montreal in November 1775. General Guy Carleton, governor general of Canada, escaped to Quebec City. The second attack was led by Colonel Benedict Arnold. Montgomery's forces joined with Arnold and his men and they attacked Quebec City on December 31 but were defeated by Carleton. Another American attack, also aimed at Quebec, failed at Trois-Rivières in June 1776.

PART TWO: EVENTS FROM 1760 UNTIL AFTER THE WAR OF 1812

Chapter 5: Between Wars

1.   For more information, see George A. Cuthbertson, *Freshwater: A History and a Narrative of the Great Lakes.* Toronto: Macmillan Co. of Canada, 1931; Harlan H. Hatcher, *Lake Erie.* Indianapolis, IN: Bobbs-Merrill, 1945; Fred Landon, *Lake Huron.* Indianapolis, IN: Bobbs-Merrill, 1944; James C. Mills, *Our Inland Seas: Their Shipping and Commerce for Three Centuries.* Cleveland, OH: Freshwater Press Inc., 1976; Milo M. Quaife, *Lake Michigan.* Indianapolis, IN: Bobbs-Merrill, 1944.

2.   K.R. Macpherson, "List of Vessels Employed on British Naval Service on the Great Lakes, 1755-1875" in *Ontario History*, Vol. 55, 1963.

3.   The Provincial Marine, an adjunct of the British Army, was a gathering of all naval assets under one name (Provincial Marine), at least on paper. These assets would include the dockyards at York, Detroit, Carleton etc., the vessels and the crew. The vessels were manned by soldiers, through officered by Royal Navy officers. The purpose was to provide transportation, keep lines of communication open and generally serve the needs of the British Army. As such, it actually was a branch of the army.

   Originally, the Provincial Marine was established under Captain Joshua Loring RN (in Massachusetts before the American Revolutionary War) and his successor Captain Alexander Grant RN, appointed Naval Superintendent to replace Loring who had been injured. It ceased to exist in the spring of 1813 when the Royal Naval took over. Some historians trace the founding of the Royal Canadian Navy back to the Provincial Marine. For more information, see James C. Mills, *Our Inland Seas: Their Shipping and Commerce for Three Centuries.*

4.   The attack at Mackinac took place at Fort Mackinac (present Mackinaw City, Michigan) on June 4, 1763. The British had occupied the fort in 1761 and only thirty-five British soldiers occupied is at the time. Also living there were their families, some remaining French fur traders and hangers-on. The local Ojibwe staged a game outside the fort, somewhat like lacrosse with the visiting Sauk and the soldiers watched the game, as they had done on previous occasions. When the ball was sent through the open gate of the fort, the team rushed after it into the fort, (ostensibly to retrieve the ball) and were then handed weapons by the Indian women who had smuggled them into the fort in their clothing and blankets. About fifteen

men of the garrison were killed in the struggle and five more were later executed, Adapted from http://en.wikipedia.org/wiki/Pontiac's°Rebellion, accessed Nov. 30, 2006.

5.   The British around this time had three big fleets of warships known as the White Fleet, the Red Fleet and the Blue Fleet. John Schank became admiral of the Blue Fleet.

6.   These very large rowing boats were used for carrying men and supplies and sometimes were fitted with sails.

7.   Arthur Britton Smith, *Legend of the Lake: the 22-gun Brig-sloop Ontario. 1780.* Kingston, ON: Quarry Press, 1997.

8.   Harlan Hatcher, *Lake Erie,* 1944.

9.   Sir William Johnson, born c. 1715 in Ireland, came to North America in 1738 to oversee an estate in the Mohawk Valley of New York, acquired by his uncle, Vice-Admiral Sir Peter Warren. With capital supplied by his naval uncle and his own astute business skills, he acquired considerable land and his shop served as a supply centre for trading goods. His success ultimately led to involvement in public affairs. In 1755, Edward Braddock, commander-in-chief in North America, selected Johnson to become the "superintendent of Northern Indians" with responsibility of managing relations between the Six Nations and their dependent tribes. It was Johnson who negotiated peace with Pontiac in 1766. Over time he acquired a considerable amount of land, much of the purchase being First Nations land. He died at Johnson Hall (Johnstown, NY) in 1774. Adapted from the Dictionary of Canadian Biography Online (Julian Gwyn) at http://www.biographi.ca/EN/ShowBio.asp?BioId=36096&query, accessed on Nov. 9, 2006.

10.   John Askin (1738-1815) was of Irish origin. He lived at Detroit for several years and is best remembered for his prolific letters.

11.   John Jacob Astor was born on Baden, Germany, in 1763. He learned English while working for one of his brothers in London, England. Astor went to New York to join another brother, arriving there in 1784 just after the end of the Revolutionary War. He started a fur goods shop there in the late 1780s. By 1800 he had become one of the leading figures in the fur trade in the United States. An able cultivator of political support, he established the American Fur Company in 1808 and later formed subsidiaries: the Pacific Fur Company and the Southwest Fur Company.

The trading post, Fort Astoria (1811), at the mouth of the Columbia River, was the first United States community on the Pacific coast. Astor had financed the overland Astor Expedition in 1810-12 to reach the outpost. In 1822, he established the Astor House on Mackinac Island for the reformed American Fur Company, making the island a metropolis of the fur trade. By 1834, he was focusing on Manhattan real estate. After his retirement, he spent the rest of his life as a patron of culture, supporting ornithologist John James Audubon and writer Edgar Alan Poe among others. When he died in 1848, Astor was the wealthiest person in the United States. Adapted from http://en.wikipedia.org/wiki/John°Jacob°Astor, accessed on Nov. 9, 2006.

12.　F. Clever Bald, "The United States Shipyard on the River Rouge" in *Inland Seas*, Vol. 6 (2 parts), 1946.

13.　The surrender of Detroit was a non-event. By Jay's Treaty (1794) the lands of America that had been occupied by the British (which included Detroit) were to be turned over to the Americans. Britain moved her men and assets to Amhertsburg (Fort Malden). By June, 1796, all was ready for removal, and on the second of June, George Beckwith, Adjutant General at Quebec, signed the order to the various commanders at the forts to evacuate immediately.

On the eleventh of July, Colonel England, the portly commander of Detroit, ordered the British flag hauled down, and marched out, transferring his troops to the new quarters at Amherstburg. For more information see Cuthbertson, *Freshwater*, 1931.

Chapter 6: Events Leading Up to the War of 1812

1.　Henry Clay (1777-1852), politician and lawyer, was the ninth US Secretary of State. The founder and leader of the Whig Party, he represented Kentucky in both the House of Representatives and the Senate. He became known as the "Great Compromiser" because of his success in brokering compromises on the slavery issue, particularly in 1820 and 1850. In 1957, a Senate committee named Clay as one of the five greatest senators in American history. Adapted from http://en.wikipedia.org/wiki/Henry°Clay, accessed on Nov. 14, 2006.

2.　Isaac Brock, born in 1769 in Guernsey, died in battle at Queenston Heights, Upper Canada, on Oct. 13, 1812. His military experience was mainly linked to the 49th Foot, which he joined in Barbados after having been an ensign in the 8th Foot in England.

When the 49th Foot was ordered to Canada in 1802, Lieutenant-Colonel Brock was part of the regiment. Brock was promoted to colonel in 1805, and about the same time went home on leave. While back in England, there was mounting apprehension of war with the United States and he decided to cut his leave short and return to his post.

The United States declared war on June 18, 1812, and on July 12, US Brigadier General William Hull invaded Canada along the Detroit Frontier. Brock, with the assistance of the Shawnee Chief Tecumseh, successfully held the fort at Amhertsburg and Hull surrendered Detroit and his army, with 35 guns and other stores that were very useful.

The chief threat was now on the Niagara Peninsula. Brock's problem was how to defend a long border line with inadequate forces, while always uncertain as to where the Americans might strike. Before daylight on the 13th, gunfire from the direction of Queenston announced that an attack was in progress. Brock rode hard towards the scene of action. Realizing the importance of evicting the American Captain John Ellis Wool from his position on the heights above Queenston, Brock collected troops nearby and led them up the slope on foot. At this moment, Brock, at six-foot-two and a splendid target, fell victim to an enemy sharpshooter.

Initially, Brock was buried at Fort George. Today the Brock Monument, a lofty column, dominates the battlefield where Brock fell at Queenston Heights. Adapted from http://www.biographi.ca/EN/ShowBio.asp?Bioid=36410&query, accessed on Nov. 14, 2006.

3.   Isaac Brock's quote is from Pierre Berton's *The Invasion of Canada, 1812–1813*. Toronto: McClelland & Stewart, 1980. He credits E.A. Cruikshank's *"Documents Relating to the Invasion of the Niagara Peninsula by the United States Army Commanded by General Jacob Brown in July and August, 1814, No. 33*, Niagara-on-the-Lake, Niagara Historical Society Publications, 1920," saying it is part of Brock's speech on opening the legislature. There is no date given, but it would have been in 1812.

4.   James Monroe (1758-1831) was born in Virginia and, like his parents, he was a slaveholder. In 1790, he was elected United States Senator. From 1794 to 1796, he was minister to France and later would help negotiate the Louisiana Purchase. In 1816 he was elected fifth president on the Republican ticket and re-elected in 1820.

Monroe is probably best known for what became known as the Monroe Doctrine. Delivered in his message to Congress in 1823, he proclaimed that the Americas should be free from future European colonization and free from European interference in sovereign countries' affairs. It stipulated the United States' intention to stay neutral in European wars and wars between European powers and their colonies. Any interference with independent countries in the Americas would be considered hostile acts towards the United States. Adapted from http://www.whitehouse.gov/history/presidents/jm5.html and http://en.wikipedia.org/wiki/James°Monroe, both accessed on Nov. 14, 2006.

5. James Madison (1751-1836) was the fourth president of the United States, serving in office from 1809 to 1817. Prior to that he had been President Jefferson's Secretary of State. Out of his leadership came the development of the Republican, or Jeffersonian, Party. On June 1, 1812, President Madison asked Congress to declare war against Britain, thus initiating what became known, in Canada, as the War of 1812. Adapted from http://www.whitehouse.gov/history/presidents/jm4.html, accessed on Nov. 14, 2006.

6. John Calhoun (1782-1850) was a congressman and a vice-president of the United States in 1824. He was known as one of the "war hawks" along with Henry Clay.

7. Isaac Chauncey (1772-1840) was born in Connecticut and served in the merchant marine as a young man. He received his first command at 19 years of age. In 1807, Captain Chauncey took command of the Navy Yard at Brooklyn, and when, in 1812, war was declared against Britain, he was sent to the Great Lakes to expand and head up the US naval forces there. He superintended the construction of a fleet on Lake Ontario and led naval actions against the British, including the attack on York in 1813. Adapted from http://www.history.navy.mil/photos/pers-us/uspers-c/i-chaunc.htm, accessed on Nov. 9, 2006.

8. James Fenimore Cooper: *Ned Myers; or, A Life Before the Mast.* Annapolis, MD: The Naval Institute Press, 1989, reprint.

9. Jacques-Yves Cousteau (1910-1997) was a French naval officer, explorer, ecologist, filmmaker, photographer and researcher who studied the sea and all forms of life in water. In his ship *Calypso* he visited the most interesting waters of the planet, and produced many books and films. Adapted from http://en.wikipedia.org/wiki/Jacques°Yves°Cousteau, accessed on Nov. 14, 2006.

Chapter 7: Declaration of War

1.　The shipyards at Erie obtained most of its munitions from Pittsburg and some from New York and Boston. However, records do not indicate the source of these guns.

2.　Henry Adams, *History of the United States of America*. New York: C. Scribner's Sons, 1889–1891.

3.　Pierre Berton in *The Invasion of Canada* refers to Isaac Brock's disenchantment. He cites a reference to E.A. Cruickshank, *Documents Relating to the Invasion*.

4.　"Franked" is a term used by postal services internationally for hundreds of years. It generally refers to a mark or signature on an envelope indicating that the sender does not have to pay postage.

5.　"Cutting-out" is a naval term meaning to capture, usually by stealth, of a vessel that is anchored offshore or perhaps left unattended for a few hours.

Chapter 8: A Shipbuilder's War

1.　Captain Andrew Gray was killed by an American sharpshooter in May 1813 during a British attack on Sacket's Harbor.

2.　The names of ships were changed frequently and sometimes the reason is not known. It seems to have been customary in the Royal Navy to never name a ship after a living monarch or high official. Perhaps it was considered back luck, but that is only a speculation. Cuthbertson, in *Freshwater*, says that the name was changed to *Wolfe* at Prevost's special request — possibly he was superstitious. Incidentally, the name *Wolfe* was changed again in 1814 to the *Montreal*. Keeping track of these names is very challenging.

3.　Taken from W.A.B. Douglas, "The Anatomy of Naval Incompetence," in *Ontario History*, Vol. 71. 1979.

4.　Author's Note: Writers have blamed the American soldiers for looting and arson. Others blame "disaffected" settlers. There is general agreement that what today we would call "fifth columnists" and "agents provocateurs" were in Upper Canada before and during the war. Whether they were free agents or planted by the US government has never even been investigated to my knowledge.

5. Robert Malcolmson in *HMS Detroit: The Battle for Lake Erie* (St. Catharines, ON: Vanwell Publishing, 1990) refers to a brief "quasi war" with France in 1800 and a lengthier war against the "pirates" of Tripoli in 1804, referred to as the Barbary War.

6. Letter from William Jones (American Secretary of the Navy) to Commodore Isaac Chauncey, January 27, 1813. USNA, M149, 10:231.

7. A "camel" was nothing more than a big box that was lowered (sunk) alongside the ship (one on each side) and the two tied together under the ship. Then it was pumped out and as it rose in the water, it lifted the ship as well. The idea is still used in salvage operations.

8. "First-rate" is a naval term from Britain, indicating the number of guns on a warship. A first-rater would have more than 110 guns.

Chapter 9: The Lake Ontario Theatre in 1813-14

1. Letter from Commodore James Yeo to the Governor General Sir George Prevost, December 2, 1813, NAC, RG8, 731:178.

2. John Strachan (1778-1807) was born in Aberdeen, Scotland, and arrived in Upper Canada in 1799, fresh out of university. In his early days he taught the "up-and-coming" generation of prominent young men, first in Kingston and then in Cornwall. He was ordained as a deacon in the Church of England in 1803, married the widow of fur trader Andrew McGill in 1807, and in 1812 he and his family moved to York where he showed considerable leadership during the War of 1812. A member of the Family Compact, he later became Bishop Strachan. He founded Trinity College in Toronto in 1851. For more information, see Robert C. Lee, *The Canada Company and the Huron Tract, 1826–1853: Personalities, Profits and Politics*. Toronto: Natural Heritage, 2004.

3. Franklin B. Hough, *History of Jefferson County in the State of New York from the Earliest Time to the Present Time*. [microform] Albany, NY: J. Munsell; Waterown, NY: Sterling & Riddell, 1854. Sacket's Harbor is in Jefferson County.

4. Dr. William "Tiger" Dunlop (1792–1848) born in Greenock, Scotland. Known for his colourful personality, he was a medical doctor, the

Canada Company's appointed Warden of the Forests and a politician. He is buried in Goderich, Ontario. For more on his life, see R.C. Lee, *The Canada Company and the Huron Tract, 1826–1853*.

5.   Letter from Commodore Isaac Chauncey to General Jacob Brown, August 10, 1814, from Chauncey's Letterbook. In the British navy at the time, whenever an officer had to write a letter or a report, his secretary usually prepared it by hand. A copy was made, also by hand, and kept in a "Letterbook," thus available in case of queries from those higher up, and also available to historians.

6.   Captain Stephen Decatur was a hero in the US Navy, primarily for actions at Tripoli in the Barberry Wars and in the War of 1812 on the Atlantic. He never left Washington for Sacket's Harbor, as Isaac Chauncey began to take action and carry out his responsibilities.

7.   The frigate *Psyche* was launched on December 25, 1814. This ship was built at Chatham Dockyard, England, and sent to Canada "in frame," carried up the St. Lawrence in pieces and assembled at Kingston. Another frigate and two brigs were sent out in the same manner, but (chiefly because of the strain on the overtaxed St. Lawrence facilities) this was the only ship sent up to the Lakes. C.P. Stacey, "The Ships of the British Squadron on Lake Ontario, 1812-14," in *Canadian Historical Review*, Vol. 34, Dec. 4, 1953.

8.   John M. Duncan, *Travels Through Part of the United States and Canada in 1818 and 1819*. Glasgow: Hurst, Robinson & Co., 1823.

9.   Much of this information is from Walter Havighurst, *The Long Ships Passing: the Story of the Great Lakes*. New York: Macmillan Co., 1942.

Chapter 10: Comments on the Battle of Lake Erie

1.   Letter from Commodore O.H. Perry to the Secretary of the Navy, September 13, 1813, taken from A. Bowen, The *Naval Monument: Containing Official and other Accounts of all the Battles Fought Between the Navies of the United States and Great Britain during the Late War, and an Account of the War with Algiers*. Boston: sold by Cummings and Hilliard, 1816.

2.   Ibid.

3.   Author's Note: Various authors say "teenagers" were among the Canadian fleet and one writer mentions two men of African descent, but

nobody truly knows. After all this was the big day! They had been building ships for months. Someone shouts, "Hey! The ships are leaving. Let's get on board!" That's probably how it happened. One writer tells of some Canadians deserting and sailing off to join the Americans. In general, nobody knows what actually happened.

4.   Fred M. Delano, "A Legend of Old Fort Malden," published in the *Detroit Free Press*, January 1, 1879, as included in Hamish A. Leach, *The Founding of Fort Amherstberg (Malden) Along the Detroit Frontier*. First published in 1796, it was reprinted in Houston by the Veldt Protea Institute in 1984.

Chapter 11: Disaffection

1.   Background for this chapter was gleaned largely from Morris Zaslow (ed.), *The Defended Border; Upper Canada and the War of 1812*. Toronto: Macmillan Co. of Canada, 1964, see chapter entitled, "A study of Diasaffection in Upper Canada in 1812-1815" by Ernest A. Cruikshank.

Chapter 12: Negotiations for Peace

1.   The negotiations took place at Ghent in Belgium from August 7 to December 24, 1814. The five American negotiators included: John Quincy Adams, James Bayard, Henry Clay, Albert Gallatin and Jonathan Russell.

2.   Alfred T. Mahan, *Sea Power in its Relations to the War of 1812*. Boston: Little, Brown, 1905.

3.   Ibid.

4.   Herbert Agar, *The Price of Union* (2nd edition). Boston: Houghton Mifflin, 1966.

Chapter 13: The Saga of the Nancy

1.   Writers have various durations for McDouall's trip. E.A. Cruikshank in "An Episode in the War of 1812: The Story of the Schooner "Nancy," *Ontario History*, Vol. 9, 1910, says, "...he left Nottawasaga on April 25...he arrived at Mackinac on May 18." Apparently in a letter Prevost wrote to Lord Bathurst, he says "nineteen days." This letter is also quoted by Cruickshank.

2.   Taken from a report written by Lt. Daniel Turner to Captain A. Sinclair, July 24, 1814, and reproduced in Cruikshank, "An Episode in the War of

1812," in *Ontario History*. Most of the information about the capture of these two schooners comes from a detailed report written by Lt. A.H. Bulger RN to Lt. Col. McDouall, Sept. 7, 1814, also reproduced by Cruikshank.

3. Taken from Elsie McLeod Jury, "U.S.S. Tigress — H.M.S. Confiance, 1813-1831," in *Inland Seas*, Vol. 28, 1964.

4. The letter from John Richardson, dated, Sept. 23, 1789, is quoted by several writers without saying to whom it is addressed. It might be that he was writing to his head office in Montreal. Taken from Cruikshank, "An Episode in the War of 1812."

5. Ibid.

6. Ibid.

7. The quotes attributed to various members of the Askin family are from Milo M. Quaif (ed.) *The Askin Papers*, Detroit Public Library Commission, 2 Volumes, 1928-31. A "Moccocka" identified in John Askin's letter, is a container made of birchbark, and used for maple sugar. This sugar was probably the first "manufactured" article traded by the Natives to the white man.

Chapter 14: The Story of the HMS Lawrence

1. Point Frederick is at Kingston, at the site of the Royal Navy Dockyard, see the sketch map of Kingston, 1812, page 72.

2. Author of this quote was not identified..

3. Author's Note: The *Victory*, Horatio Nelson's ship at the Battle of Trafalgar, is the most famous ship in Britain's history, bar none. The ship still exists, as a tourist destination and memorial, at Portsmouth, England. I was on it, examining how it was put together, and making a few measurements.

4. Letter from Sir James Yeo to John Croker, First Secretary of the Admiralty, dated Oct. 26, 1814, as quoted in J. Douglas Stewart and Ian E, Wilson, *Heritage Kingston*. Kingston, ON: Queen's University (exhibition book), 1973.

5. Excerpt from David Wingfield's diary, taken from David Wingfield, "Four Years on the Lakes of Canada in 1813, 1814, 1815 and 1816 by a Naval Officer under the Command of Sir James Lucas Yeo Kt Commodore

and Commander in Chief of H.M. Ships and vessels of war employed on the Lakes. Also nine months as Prisoner of War In the United States of America," Library and Archives Canada, M6.24, F18.

6.   The Rush-Bagot Agreement was negotiated by Acting United States Secretary of State Richard Rush and the British Minister to Washington Sir Charles Bagot. While the agreement addressed naval disarmament of the Great Lakes, the United States and Britain continued to build land fortifications along the border for the next half century. Ultimately, the treaty laid the basis for a demilitarized boundary between the US and the Canadas in the period following the War of 1812. Adapted from http://en.wikipedia.org/wiki/Rush-Bagot°Treaty, accessed Nov. 15, 2006.

7.   The author is indebted to Ozzie Schenk for providing him with a copy of "The Silent St. Lawrence" by C.H.J. Snider. Printed by Rous and Mann Press Ltd., Toronto, not dated. For greater detail on the ships of the Great Lakes during the period, see Robert Malcolmson, *Warships of the Great Lakes, 1754–1834*. London: Caxton Editions, 2003.

Part Three:
Shipbuilding in a Wilderness Setting

Chapter 15: Ship Construction in the Early 19th Century

1.   H.C. Inches, *The Great Lakes Wooden Shipbuilding Era*,[Vermillion?] oh: s. n., 1962.

2.   John Spurr, "Sir Robert Hall (1778-1818)" in *Queen's Archives*, Vol. 29, Feb. 20, 1980. Note that no copper was used in Upper Canada at this time. Spurr's reference is to another ship and venue entirely. However, ships constructed in Britain were coppered.

3.   Inches, *The Great Lakes Wooden Ship Building Era*.

4.   Ibid.

5.   Ibid.

6.   John E. Horsely, *Tools of the Maritime Trades*. Newton Abbot, UK: David and Charles, 1978.

7.   Rudyard Kipling (1865-1936) was born in Bombay, India, educated in England and spent parts of his adult life living in India, in Vermont, USA, and finally back in England. He was one of the most popular writers in England, in both prose and verse, in the late 19th and early 20th centuries. In 1907, he was awarded the Nobel Prize for Literature, the first English language writer to receive the prize. He is well-known for his *Jungle Book* stories for children and his novel *Kim* (1901).In 1922, Kipling was asked by a University of Toronto civil engineering professor to assist in developing a dignified "obligation" ceremony for its graduating engineering students. He did, and today engineering students all across Canada, and in some places in the USA, are presented with an iron ring at the ceremony as a reminder of their obligation to society. Adapted from http://en. wikipedia.org/wiki/ Rudyard°Kipling, accessed Jan. 12, 2007.

8.   Stanley T. Spicer, *Masters of Sail: The Era of Square-rigged Vessels in the Maritime Provinces*. Toronto: Ryerson Press, 1968.

9.   Henry Wadsworth Longfellow (1802-1882), an American poet, born in Portland, Maine. He was descended from the Longfellow family that came to the New England Colonies in 1676. His works include "Paul Revere's Ride," The Song of Hiawatha," "Evangeline" and the famous poem "The Village Blacksmith" (1841). In 1836, Longfellow became a professor of French and Spanish at Harvard University, and remained there for the rest of his life. He began publishing poetry in 1839. Adapted from http://en.wikipedia.org/wiki/Longfellow, accessed Jan. 12, 2007.

10.   Letter from Sir James Yeo to Lord Melville at Brompton, near Chatham, England, dated May 30, 1815. Apparently, when news reached Kingston that the war was over, many of the British returned home immediately Some visited Sacket's as tourists, on the way to Boston or New York.

11.   Quote from Lieut. David Wingfield, RN, taken from his diary, "Four Years on the Lakes of Canada 1813–816 by a Naval officer under the command of Sir James Lucas Yeo Kt Commodore and Commander in Chief of H.M. Ships and vessels of War employed on the Lakes. Also nine months as Prisoner of War in the United States of America," Library and Archives Canada, M6.24, F18.

12.   Theodore Roosevelt, *The Naval War of 1812, or, The History of the United States Navy During the Last War with Great Britain*. New York: G.P. Putnam's Sons, 1882.

Part Four: Commercial Sail on the Lakes Until the Early 1900s

Chapter 16: Schooner Days, Anecdotal Material and Commercial Sail

1.   Taken from one of C.H.J. Snider's articles, author not identified.

2.   The Niagara Portage Road ran from the Niagara River opposite Lewiston, New York to Lake Erie near present-day Fort Erie, Ontario.

3.   "Revenue cutter" was an early name for vessels that ensured taxes on cargo were paid. They were operated by the early equivalent of the IRS.

4.   Early Chicago had no harbour, and the sediment deposited at the mouth of the Chicago River built up a sandbar that prevented vessels from entering the river much of the time.

5.   C.H.J. Snider, "Schooner Days," a series of 1301 articles in the *Toronto Evening Telegram*, now available from the Archives of Ontario. All quotes attributed to Snider are from this source.

6.   Fore-and-aft rig means that the sails were rigged to spread parallel to a fore-and-aft line (the centre line) of the vessel. The alternative is "square-rigged," which some considered better for going downwind, but which never proved to be better in the restricted waters of the Great Lakes.

7.   Both Captain Bradley and Boscawen were part of the British Army that occupied Oswego in 1755. Bradley's comment clearly indicates that as early as 1755, the fore-and-aft rig was found to be superior.

8.   For more information, see Arthur Britton Smith, *Legend of the Lake: The 22-gun Brig Sloop Ontario, 1780*. Kingston, ON: Quarry Press, 1958.

9.   For more information, see James C. Mills, *Our Inland Seas Their Shipping and Commerce for Three Centuries*. Cleveland, OH: Freshwater Press, 1976.

10.   A knot is one nautical mile per hour.

11.   John Brandt Mansfield, *History of the Great Lakes*, 2 Vols., Chicago, 1918. Reprinted, J.H. Beers, *The Saga of the Great Lakes*. Toronto: Coles Publishing, 1980.

12. Walter Havighurst, *The Long Ships Passing*, 1942.

13. See the *Annual Report of the Lake Carriers' Association*, 1913.

14. *The Signal* (Goderich, Ontario), Nov. 20, 1913.

15. *The Collingwood Bulletin*, Dec. 4, 1913.

16. Quote attributed to G. Mann is taken from D.W. Thomson, *Men and Meridians*: The History of Surveying and mapping in Canada. Ottawa: Roger Duhamel, Queen's Printer, 1966–69.

17 Quote attributed to Capt. J.G. Boulton is taken from D.W. Thompson, *Men and Meridians*.

Chapter 17: Fur Trade on the Lakes

1. Antoine Laumet Cadillac, born in France in 1658, was a fur trader and military officer. Of obscure origins, he gave himself a noble title, de Lamothe Cadillac, and was successful in promoting himself to wealth and positions of authority. A protégé of Frontenac, he was commandant at Michilimackinac from 1693 to 1697 and was involved in the fur trade. When a glut of furs led to closing out trade with the west, he established a settlement at Detroit in 1701 as a way of preventing English expansion and, at the same time, control trade with western First Nations. In 1710, he was removed from command when it became obvious that he was in the process of creating an empire for himself.

He was governor of Louisiana from 1710 to 1717, but was soon in difficulty with officials there. He went back to France in 1718 and lived out his life as governor of Castelsarrasin, where he died in 1730. Adapted from http://www.thecanadianencyclopedia.com/index.cfm?PgNm=TCE&Params=A1ARTA0001161, accessed on Dec. 8, 2006.

2. Pierre-Esprit Radisson (1636-1710) was a French-born explorer and fur trader. Along with his brother-in-law, Médard Chouart des Groseilliers (1618-c. 1696), he explored the area around Lakes Superior and Michigan. In 1668, they travelled to Hudson Bay on behalf of a group of English merchants (the nucleus of the Hudson's Bay Company). They made a number of fur-trading expeditions there until 1675. From Katharine Barber (ed.), *The Canadian Oxford Dictionary* (Toronto: Oxford University Press, 1998).

3. Daniel Greysolon, Sieur du Lhut (c. 1639-1710), a French soldier and explorer, was the first European known to have visited the location of

present-day Duluth, Minnesota, and the headwaters of the Mississippi River near Grand Rapids, Minnesota. He arrived to settle rivalries between two Native nations, the Ojibwa and the Dakota, in order to advance fur trading missions in the area.

Subsequently, Du Lhut established fortifications to defend French interests at Fort Caministigoyan at the mouth of the Kaministiquia River (Thunder Bay, Ontario). Seemingly the onset of gout curtailed his activities as an explorer, and he spent his last 15 years uneventfully in Montreal. From his name comes the name of the City of Duluth. Adapted from http://en.wikipedia.org/wiki/Daniel°Greysolon%2C°Sieur°du°Lhut and http://en.wikipedia.org/wiki/Duluth%2C°Minnesota, both accessed on Dec. 8, 2006.

4.   For more information on the fur trade and, in particular, on the North West Company, see Jean Morrison, *Superior Rendezvous-Place: Fort William in the Canadian Fur Trade.* Toronto: Natural Heritage Books, 2001.

5.   Jay's Treaty was signed on Nov. 19, 1794, by the US and Britain. It was named for John Jay, a US chief justice and a signatory. A primarily commercial agreement, it was intended to settle disputes that threatened war between the two countries.

The treaty marks the revival of arbitration in international relations. Adapted from http://www.thecanadianencyclopedia.com/index.cfm?PgNm=TCE&Params=A1ARTA0004114 (Stuart R.J. Sutherland), accessed on Dec. 8, 2006.

Chapter 18: Fishing on the Lakes

1.   John Johnston, *Account of Lake Superior 1792-1807*, 1807. An electronic transcription. MFTP #0037.

2.   Hazel C. Mathews, *Oakville and the Sixteen: The History of an Ontario Port.* Toronto: University of Toronto Press, 1965.

3.   Ibid.

4.   Anna Brownell Jameson, *Winter Studies and Summer Rambles in Canada,* Toronto: Thomas Nelson, 1943.

5.   Ibid.

6.   Quote attributed to Rev. James Evans taken from William Sherwood, *The Bruce Beckons*. Toronto: University of Toronto Press, 1952. For more on James Evans, see Roger Burford Mason, *Travels in the Shining Island*, Toronto: Natural Heritage Books, 1996.

7.   Norman Robertson, *History of the County of Bruce: And of the Minor Municipalities Therein*. Toronto: William Briggs, 1906.

8.   John Galt (1779–1939) was born in Irvine, Scotland. Known as a novelist, adventurer and lobbyist, he claimed that the Canada Company (a British financed land settlement company that acquired thousands of acres of unopened land in Upper Canada to sell to new arrivals) was his idea. He actively and successfully promoted its establishment in 1826. Galt became the first commissioner of the Company but was recalled to England in 1829. Galt is recognized as the founder of Guelph (April 1827). John and Elizabeth (Tilloch) Galt's youngest son, (Sir) Alexander Tilloch Galt, was a member of the legislature of Canada (1849-50s; 1853-67), a "Father of Confederation" and Canada's first High Commissioner to London.

9.   Robert A. Sinclair, *Winds Over Lake Huron: Chronicles in the Life of a Great Lakes Mariner*. Hicksville, NY: Exposition Press, 1960.

10.   Bill Bermingham went on to found the Bermingham Marine Construction Company that operated out of Hamilton, Ontario, and functions today as Bermingham Construction Limited. They own one barge called *Spike B*, named after the founder.

11.   H Ted Gozzard's company, a family-operated business has a long history of building pleasure boats in Huron County. As well as luxury sailing yachts, the company also builds a small number of trawlers in the 50-foot range. His sailing vessels, known as "Gozzards" or "H.T. Gozzards," are found around the world, wherever serious sailors are cruising. The Gozzard name is synonymous with quality and excellent workmanship. Ted Gozzard was the principal designer of an earlier well-known type of sailing yacht, the Bayfield, many of which are also found worldwide.

Chapter 19: The Timber Droghers

1.   The terms "lumber droghers" and "timber droghers" are used interchangeably.

2.   The quote attributed to Sir Richard Bonnycastle is taken from James P. Barry, *Georgian Bay the Sixth Great Lake*. Toronto: Clarke, Irwin, 1968.

3.   Quote attributed to Stewart Holbrook (*Iron Brew: A Century of American Ore and Steel*, 1939) is also from James P. Barry.

4.   Harlan Hatcher, *Lake Erie*, 1945.

Chapter 20: Other Commercial Sail, Ore Carriers and Stone Hookers

1.   There were early copper mines on the "copper peninsula" now known as Keweenaw Peninsula. Also pure copper was found on Isle Royale, Thunder Bay. Silver ores frequently are found with copper ores in geological formations. One of the largest silver strikes was at Siver Islet, a small island in Lake Superior. For more information on Silver Islet, see Elinor Barr, *Silver Islet: Striking it Rich in Lake Superior*. Toronto: Natural Heritage Books, 1988, reprinted 1995.

2.   Henry Rowe Schoolcraft (1793-1864) was an American geographer, geologist and ethnologist. His ethnological work began in 1822 when he was appointed Indian agent at Sault Ste. Marie, Michigan. Married to Jane Johnson, daughter of an Irish fur trader and an Ojibwe woman, he learned the Ojibwe language and lore of the tribe. In 1832, he went back to the upper reaches of the Mississippi River, explored the region and made the first accurate map of the Lake District around western Lake Superior. Also at this time he discovered the true headwaters of the Mississippi River. Adapted from http://en.wikipedia.org/wiki/Henry°Schoolcraft, accessed on Dec. 8, 2006.

3.   Regular trains run on tracks made of rolled steel. A strap railway uses wooden beams. The railway runs on a steel strap fastened on these beams. This seems to be restricted to mining and ore handling, where the rail line is only needed for a relatively short period of time and where cars are lighter in weight as compared to ordinary rail cars.

4.   The story of the *Bruno* was provided by Peter White, whose father had boarded with Captain Peters' family in Toronto. Additional information on the story of the shipwreck of the *Bruno* and the *Louisa* was adapted from http://www.hhpl.on.ca/GreatLakes/Wrecks/details.asp?ID=17554, accessed on Jan. 19, 2007.

Bibliography

PART ONE: THE ERA OF FRENCH CONTROL ON
THE GREAT LAKES, 1678–1760

Primary Sources:
(i) Books

Hennepin, Father Louis, *A New Discovery of a Vast Country in America....* First
    published London, 1698. Reprinted Toronto: Coles Publishing Co., 1974.

Secondary Sources:
(ii) Books

Cuthbertson, George A., *Freshwater: A History and a Narrative of the Great
    Lakes.* Toronto: Macmillan of Canada, 1931.

Hatcher, Harlan H., *Lake Erie.* Indianapolis, IN: Bobbs-Merrill, 1945.

Landon, Fred, *Lake Huron.* Indianapolis, IN: Bobbs-Merrill, 1944.

MacLean, Harrison John, *The Fate of the Griffon.* Toronto: Griffin House, 1974.

Marshall, O.H., *The Building and Voyage of the Griffon in 1679* [microform].
    Publication of the Buffalo Historical Society, Bigelow Bros. 1879.

Porter, Peter A., *How Lake Commerce Began: La Salle's Visits to the Niagara*
    (Niagara Falls, NY: 1914?.

Quaife, Milo M., *Lake Michigan.* Indianapolis, IN: Bobbs-Merrill, 1944.

Quimby, George Irving, *Indian Culture and European Trade Goods: The
    Archaeology of the Historic Period in the Western Great Lakes Region.*
    Madison, WI: University of Wisconsin Press, 1966. Reprinted
    Westport, CT: Greenwood Press, 1978.

Remington, Cyrus Kingsbury, *The Ship-yard of the Griffon: A Brigantine
    Built by René Robert Cavelier, Sieur de La Salle, in the Year 1679,
    Above the Falls of Niagara.* Buffalo, NY: J.W. Clement, 1891.

Severance, Frank H., *An Old Frontier of France: The Niagara Region and
    Adjacent Lakes Under French Control.* 2 vols. New York: Dodd, Mead,
    1917.

Swayze, Fred, *Tonty of the Iron Hand.* Toronto: Ryerson Press, 1957.

(ii) Journals/Newspapers

Baker, Wallace J., "On Manitoulin Island" in *Inland Seas*, 1947.

Fleming, Roy F., "The Search for La Salle's Griffon" in *Inland Seas*, Winter 1952 and Spring 1953.

_____, "First Sailor of the Upper Lakes" in *The Canadian Magazine*, August 1929.

Fox, George F., "Was This La Salle's Griffon?" in *The Beaver*, Winter 1955.

Murphy, Rowley W., "Discovery of the Wreckage of the Griffon" in *Inland Seas*, Winter 1955, Spring 1956 and Summer 1956.

Myers, Frank A., "The Manitoulin Griffon vs the Tobermory Griffon" in *Inland Seas*, Vol. 12, 1956.

Snider, C.H.J., "Further Search for the Griffon" in *Ontario History*, Vol. 44, 31 and 48, 1956.

_____, "Schooner Days" in *Toronto Telegram*, Aug. 20, 1955.

Tappenden, Richard P., "Possible Solution to the Mystery of the Griffon" in *Inland Seas*, Winter 1946.

Walsh-Sarnecki, Peggy, "Shipwreck Explorer Hires Help" in *Detroit Free Press*, Aug. 14, 2006.

Part Two: Events From 1760 Until After the War of 1812

Primary Sources

(i) Books

Bigsby, John J., *The Shoe and Canoe, or, Pictures of Travel in the Canadas: Illustrative of their Scenery and Colonial Life; With Facts and Opinions on Emigration, State Policy and Other Points of Public Interest.* London: Chapman and Hall, 1850. Reprinted New York: Paladin Press, 1969.

Bowen, Abel, *The Naval Monument, containing official and other accounts of the Battles fought between the navies of the United States and Great Britain during the late wars, and an account of the war with Algiers.* Boston: sold by Cummins and Hillard, 1816.

Duncan, John M., *Travels Through Part of the United States and Canada in 1818 and 1819.* Glasgow: Hurst, Robinson & Co., 1823.

Heriot, George, *Travels through the Canadas.* Toronto: Coles Publishing Co., 1971, first published 1807.

Hough, Franklin B., *History of Jefferson County in the State of New York from the Earliest Times to the Present Time* [microform]. Albany, NY: J. Munsell; Watertown, NY: Sterling & Riddell, 1854.

Jameson, Anna Brownell, *Winter Studies and Summer Rambles in Canada.* New York: Wiley and Putnam, 1839. First published London: Saunders and Otley, 1838.

Wingfield, David, *Four Years on the Lakes of Canada 1813-1816 by a Naval Office*, held at Library and Archives Canada, M6.24, F18.

Secondary Sources:
(i) Books

Agar, Herbert, *The Price of Union*. Boston: Riverside Press/Houghton, 1966.

Barnes, James, *Naval Actions of the War of 1812*. New York: Harper & Brothers, 1896.

Benn, Carl, *The Battle of York*. Belleville, ON: Mika, 1984.

Barry, James, *The Battle of Lake Erie, September, 1813: TheNaval Battle that Decided a Northern US Boundary*. New York: Franklin Watts Inc., 1970.

Berton, Pierre, *The Invasion of Canada*. Toronto: McClelland & Stewart, 1980.

_____, *Flames Across the Border*. Toronto: McClelland & Stewart, 1981.

Burton, Clarence Monroe (Milo M. Quaife ed.), *When Detroit Was Young*. Detroit: Burton Abstract and Title Co., 195?.

Cain, Emily, *Ghost Ships, Hamilton and Scourge; Historical Treasures from the War of 1812*. Toronto: Musson, 1983.

Chapelle, Howard I., *The History of the American Sailing Navy: The Ships and Their Devlopment*. New York: Bonanza Books, 1949.

Dobbins, W.W., *History of the Battle of Lake Erie (September 10, 1813): and Reminiscences of the Flagship "Lawrence."* Erie, PA: Ashby & Vincent, 1876.

Douglas, W.A.B., *Gunfire on the Lakes: The Naval War of 1812-1814 on the Great Lakes and Lake Champlain*. Ottawa: National Museum of Man, 1977.

Dutton, Charles J., *Oliver Hazard Perry*. New York/Toronto: Longmans, Green, 1935.

Forester, C. S., *The Age of Fighting Sail, The Story of the Naval War of 1812*. Garden City, NY: Doubleday, 1956.

Gardiner, Robert (ed.), *The Naval War of 1812*, Annapolis, MD: Naval Institute Press, 1998.

Gough, Barry M., *Fighting Sail on Lake Huron and Georgian Bay: The War of 1812 and Its Aftermath*. Annapolis, MD: Naval Institute Press, 2002.

Gough, Barry M., *Through Water, Ice and Fire: Schooner Nancy and the War of 1812*. Toronto: Dundurn Group, 2006.

Havighurst, Walter, *Three Flags at the Straits: The Forts of Mackinac*. Englewood Cliffs, NJ: Prentice-Hall, 1966.

Hitsman, M., *The Incredible War of 1812: A Military History*. Updated by Donald E. Graves. Toronto: Robin Brass Studio, 1999.

Mahan, Alfred T., *Sea Power in its Relations to the War of 1812*. Boston: Little, Brown, 1905.

Malcomson, Robert, *Lords of the Lake: The Naval War on Lake Ontario 1812–1814*. Toronto: Robin Brass Studio, 2001, c1998.

_____, *Warships of the Great Lakes, 1754–1834*. Annapolis, MD: Naval Institute Press, 2001. Reprinted London: Caxton Editions, 2003.

_____, and Thomas Malcomson, *HMS Detroit The Battle for Lake Erie*. St. Catharines, ON: Vanwell Publishing, 1990.

Parkman, Francis, *France and England in North America*. New York: Library Classics of the United States, distributed to the trade by Viking Press, 1983.

Preston, Richard A. (ed.), *Kingston Before the War of 1812: A Collection of Documents*. Toronto: Champlain Society, University of Toronto Press, 1959.

Roosevelt, Theodore, *The Naval War of 1812, Vols. 1 &2*. Part of the series *The Works of Theodore Roosevelt* (14 volumes). New York: C. Scribner, 1906–1920.

Rosenberg, Max, *The Building of Perry's Fleet on Lake Erie, 1812–1813*. Harrisburg, PA: Pennsylvania Historical and Museums Commission, 1950.

Smith, Arthur Britton, *Legend of the Lake: The 22-gun Brig-sloop "Ontario" 1780*. Kingston, ON: Quarry Press, 1997.

Snider, C.H.J., *Tarry Breeks and Velvet Garters: Sail on the Great Lakes of America*. Toronto: Ryerson Press, 1958.

_____, *The Silent St. Lawrence: An Angel of Enduring Peace*. Toronto: Rous and Mann, 1948?.

_____, *The Story of the "Nancy" and other Eighteen-Twelvers*. Toronto: McClelland & Stewart, 1926.

_____, *In the Wake of the Eighteen-Twelvers; Fights & Flights of Frigates & Fore-'n' afters in the War of 1812–1815 on the Great Lakes*. London: J. Lane; Toronto: Bell & Cockburn 1913.

Stewart, J. Douglas & Wilson, Ian E. *Heritage Kingston*. Kingston, ON: Queen's University [exhibition book], 1973

Suthren, Victor, *The War of 1812*. Toronto: McClelland & Stewart, 1999.

Zaslow, Morris (ed.), *The Defended Border: Upper Canada and the War of 1812*. Toronto: Macmillan of Canada, 1964.

(ii) Journals/Newspapers

Alford, Harold D., "Shipbuilding Days in Old Oswego" in *Inland Seas* (2 parts), 1951.

Bald, F. Clever, "The United States Shipyard on the River Rouge" in *Inland Seas*, Vol. 6 (2 parts), 1946.

Breithaupt, W.H., "Some Facts about the Schooner 'NANCY' in the War of 1812" in *Ontario History*, Vol. 23, 1926.

Cumberland, Barlow, "The Navies of Lake Ontario in the War of 1812" in *Ontario History*, Vol. 8, 1909.

Cruikshank, E.A., "Notes on the History of Shipbuilding and Navigation on Lake Ontario" in *Ontario History*, Vol. 23, 1926.

_____, "The Contest for the Command of Lake Ontario in 1814" in *Ontario History*, Vol. 21, 1924.

_____, "An Episode of the War of 1812: The Story of the Schooner 'Nancy' " in *Ontario History*, Vol. 9, 1910.

Curry, Frederick C., "Six Little Schooners" in *Inland Seas*, Vol. 2, 1946.

Douglas, W.A.B., "The Anatomy of Naval Incompetence: The Provincial Marine in Defence of Upper Canada before 1813" in *Ontario History*, Vol. 71, 1979.

Green, Ernest, "Corvettes of New France" in Ontario History, Vol. 5, 1921, 28-38.

Humphries, Charles W., "The Capture of York" in *Ontario History*, Vol. 51, 1959.

Jury, Elsie McLeod, "U.S.S. Tigress — H.M.S. Confiance, 1813-1831" in *Inland Seas*, Vol. 28, 1972.

Macpherson, K.R., "List of Vessels Employed on British Naval Service on the Great Lakes, 1755–1875" in *Ontario History*, Vol. 55, 1963.

Metcalf, Clarence, "Daniel Dobbins, Sailing Master" in *Inland Seas* (2 parts), Vol. 14.2 (1958) 88-96; Vol. 14.3 (1958) 181-196.

Metcalf, C.S., "The Battle of Lake Erie" in *Inland Seas*, Vol. 4, 1948.

Murphy, Rowley, "Resurrection at Penetanguishene" in *Inland Seas*, Vol. 10, 1954.

Preston, Richard A., "The Fate of Kingston's Warships" in *Ontario History*, Vol. 44, 1952.

Snider, C.H.J., "Schooner Days," 131 articles in the *Toronto Telegram*, now available on a CD from Archives Ontario.

Stacey, C.P., "Another Look at the Battle of Lake Erie" in *Canadian Historical Review*, Vol. 39, 1958.

_____, "The Ships of the British Squadron on Lake Ontario, 1812-14" in *Canadian Historical Review*, Vol. 34, 1953.

_____, "The War of 1812 in Canadian History" in *Ontario History*, Vol. 50, 1958.

_____, "An American Plan for a Canadian Campaign" in *Ontario History*, Vol. 46, 1941.

Stickney, Kenneth, "Logistics and Communications in the 1814 Campaign," University of Toronto, unpublished MA thesis, 1976.

Winton-Clare, C., "A Shipbuilder's War" in *Mariner's Mirror*, Vol. 29, 1943.

Wheelock, Phyllis DeKay, "Henry Eckford, American Shipbuilder" in *American Neptune*, Vol. 3, No. 3, July 1947.

PART THREE: SHIPBUILDING IN A WILDERNESS SETTING

Primary Sources:
(i) Books

Fincham, John, *A History of Naval Architecture to Which is Prefixed an Introductory Dissertation on the Application of Mathematical Science to the Art of Naval Construction*. London: Whittaker, 1850; LC Call no. VM15.F48.

Secondary Sources:
(i) Books

Abell, Westcott, Sir, *The Shipwright's Trade*. Cambridge: Cambridge University Press, 1948.

Adkins Jan, *Wooden Ship*. Brooklin, MN: WoodenBoat Publications, 2004.

Archibald, E.H.H., *The Wooden Fighting Ship in the Royal Navy*. London: Blanford Press, 1968.

Boudriot, Jean, *Le Vaisseau de 74 canons: Traite pratique d'art naval*. Grenoble, France: Éditons Des Quatre Seigneurs, 1973.

Brady, William N., *The Kedge Anchor; or, Young Sailor's Assistant*. Ottawa: Algrove Publications, 2003.

Chapman, Fredrik Henrik, *Architectura Navalis Mercatoria: A Facsimile of the Classic Eighteenth Century Treatise on Shipbuilding*. New York: Praeger, 1971, c1968.

Chapelle, Howard, *The History of American Sailing Ships*. New York: Bonanza Books, 1935.

_____, The *History of American Sailing Navy: The Ships and Their Development*. New York: Bonanza Books, 1949.

_____, *Search for Speed Under Sail, 1700–1855*. New York: Norton, 1967.

Desmond, Charles, *Wooden Ship-Building*. New York: The Rudder Publishing Company, 1919.

Dodds, James and Moore, James, *Building the Wooden Fighting Ship*. London, UK: Chatham Pub., 2005.

Goldenberg, Joseph A., *Shipbuilding in Colonial America*. Charlotteville: Published for the Mariners Museum, Newport News, Virginia, by the University Press of Virginia, 1976.

Holland, A.J., *Ships of British Oak: The Rise and Decline of Wooden Shipbuilding in Hampshire*. Newton Abbot: David and Charles, 1971.

Havigurst, Walter, *The Long Ships Passing: The Story of the Great Lakes*. New York: Macmillan, 1942.

Horseley, John E., *Tools of the Maritime Trades*. Newton Abbott: David and Charles, 1978.

Howard, Frank, *Sailing Ships of War 1400-1860*. London: Conway Maritime Press, 1979.

Inches, H.C., *The Great Lakes Wooden Shipbuilding Era*. Vermillion, OH: s.n., 1962

Landstrom, Bjorn, *The Ship*. London: Allen and Unwin, 1961.

Longridge, C. Nepean, *The Anatomy of Nelson's Ships*. London: Percival Marshal, 1955.

Manning, Samuel F., *New England Masts and the King's Broad Arrow*. Kennebuck, ME: Thomas Murphy, Publisher, 1979.

Mansfield, John B., *History of the Great Lakes*. Chicago: J.H. Beers, 1899; Cleveland: Freshwater Press, 1972.

McKay, Lauchlan *The Practical Ship-builder: Published in Original Format With Seven Large Folded Plates, With Biography of Lauchlan McKay, Master-Shipbuilder*. New York: private printing, Richard C. McKay, 1940.

Spicer, Stanley T., *Masters of Sail*. Halifax, NS: Petheric Press, 1981.

Steel David, *Elements of Mastmaking, Sailmaking and Rigging*. New York: Edward W. Sweetman, 1932.

Van Gaasbeeck, *Wooden Boat and Shipbuilding*. Chicago: Frederick Drake & Co., 1941.

Wallace, Frederick William, *Wooden Ships and Iron Men*. London: Hodder & Stoughton, 1900.

Winfield, Rif, *The 50-Gun Ship*. London: Chatham Publishing, 1997.

Woods, Virginia S., *Live Oaking: Southern Timber for Tall Ships*. Annnapolis, MD: Naval Institute Press, 1995.

(ii) Journals

Salman, R.A., "Tools of the Shipwright 1650-1925" in *Folklife*, Vol. 5, 1961.

PART FOUR: COMMERCIAL SAIL ON THE LAKES UNTIL THE EARLY 1900S

Secondary Sources
(i) Books

Askin, John, (Quaife, Milo M. ed.), *John Askin Papers*. Detroit: Detroit Public Library Commission, 1928-1931.

Barry, James P., *Georgian Bay: The Sixth Great Lake*. Toronto: Clarke, Irwin, 1968.

_____, Ships of the Great Lakes: 300 Years of Navigation. Berkeley: Howell North, 1973.

Fox, William Sherwood, *The Bruce Beckons: The Story of Lake Huron's Great Peninsula*. Toronto: University of Toronto, Press 1952.

Hamil, Fred Coyne, *The Valley of the Lower Thames, 1640–1850*. Toronto: University of Toronto Press, 1951.

Havighurst, Walter, *The Great Lakes Reader*. New York: Macmillan, 1978.

_____, *The Long Ships Passing: The Story of the Great Lakes*. New York: Macmillan, 1942.

Mansfield, John B., *History of the Great Lakes*. Chicago: J.H. Beers, 1899; Reprinted as *The Saga of the Great Lakes*. Toronto: Coles Publishing 1980.

Mathews, Hazel C., *Oakville and the Sixteen: The History of an Ontario Port*. Toronto: University of Toronto Press 1953.

Mills Judith Christine, *The Stonehook Schooner*. Toronto: Key Porter Kids, 1995.

Mills, James C., *Our Inland Seas: Their Shipping and Commerce for Three Centuries*. Cleveland, OH: Freshwater Press, 1976, c1910.

Robertson, Norman, *History of the County of Bruce: And of the Minor Municipalities Therein*. Toronto: William Briggs, 1906.

Sinclair, Robert A., *Winds Over Lake Huron: Chronicles in the Life of a Great Lakes Mariner*. Hicksville, NY: Exposition Press, 1960.

Thomson, D.W., *Men and Meridians: The History of Surveying and Mapping in Canada*. Ottawa: Roger Duhamel, Queen's Printer, 1966-69.

Young, Anna, *Off Watch: Today and Yesterday on the Great Lakes*. Toronto: Ryerson Press, 1957.

Author's Note: A group of books, written in the 1940s and known as *The American Lakes Series* are about much more than sail and contain interesting anecdotal material. They are well worth reading for anyone interested in the Great Lakes and the coastal cities. All books were published by The Bobbs-Merrill Co. of Indianapolis, Indiana. The titles include: *Lake Champlain and Lake George* (Frederick F. Van De Water), *Lake Erie* (Harlan H. Hatcher), *Lake Huron* (Fred Landon), *Lake Michigan* (Milo M. Quaife), *Lake Ontario* (Arthur Pound), *Lake Superior* (Grace Lee Nute).

Author's Note: Three books were published by J. H. Beers & Co. in 1899 and reprinted by Coles Publishing Co. Ltd in 1980. They are an excellent source of information on early shipping on the Great Lakes. However, personaly I have not found them entirely reliable on matters of naval history. The titles include: *Trading and Shipping on the Great Lakes, Adventures on the Great Lakes* and *The Saga of the Great Lakes*.

(ii) Journals/Newspapers

Barry, Paul James, "Huron and Haywood Boats" in *Yachting*, April, 1942.

———, "Mackinaw Boats & Collingwood Skiffs" in *Yachting*, Nov. 1940.

Brotherton,R.A., "The Jackson Mine and Naegaunee, Michigan" in *Inland Seas*, 1946.

Ericson, Bernard, E., "*The Evolution of the Great Lakes Ships*" in *Inland Seas*, Vol. 25.2 (1969) 91-104; Vol. 25.3 (1969) 199-212.

Gardner, James, "Classic Great Lakes Fishing Craft Is Building Project for Illinois Man" in *National Fisherman*, Feb. 1983.

Hamil, Fred Coyne, "Early Shipping and Land Transportation on the Lower Thames" in *Ontario History*, date not available.

Hunter, H.A., "Collingwood Skiffs" in GAM, Feb, 1977.

Musham, H.A., "Ships That Went Down to the Seas" in *Inland Seas*, Oct. 1945.

Odle, Thomas D., "The American Grain Trade of the Great Lakes, 1825–1873" in *Inland Seas*, 19??.

Snider, C.H.J., "Schooner Days," a series of 131 articles in the *Toronto Telegram*, now available on CD from Archives Ontario. There is much in these articles on commercial shipping and on the lives of the mariners in the days of sail.

Swanson, Roger C., "Edith Jane: A Search for the Real Mackinaw Boat" in *Wooden Boat*, 1945.

Index

About the Author

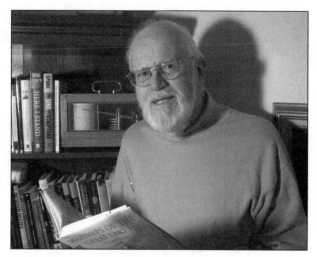

DON BAMFORD graduated from the University of Toronto in 1942 as an electrical engineer and worked for several years in the field of electronic devices for the military, atomic energy, medical and hospital applications. After a stint with the design and manufacture of small sailboats, he joined the Ontario government as an industrial consultant specializing in production efficiency and export marketing.

He retired in 1984 and immediately took up long-distance sailing. Don sailed into Lake Superior, which was the only one of the Great Lakes he hadn't previously been on, then down to the Bahamas and other Caribbean islands. In 1986, he sailed across the Atlantic from St. Petersburg, Florida, to the Hebrides and continued to sail European waters with his wife, family and friends. His wandering took him from northern Norway south to Tunisia, from Ireland to Cyprus — altogether around 25,000 miles, including every European country with a freshwater coastline except Albania. In 2000, family health problems brought an end to the sailing activities. Don sold his yacht in Devon, England, and came back to Canada.

In the early 1970s, while living and working in Chicago, Don took an interest in early sailing on the Great Lakes and researched the subject extensively, visiting many museums and historical societies in America and Europe. *Freshwater Heritage* is his third book. As well, he has had over a hundred articles on sailing and history published in magazines in Canada, the United States and the United Kingdom.

Don Bamford currently lives in London, Ontario.